NATURAL HEALING

THROUGH AYURVEDA

NATURAL HEALIING

THROUGH AYURVEDA

by Dr. Subhash Ranade

Edited by Dr. David Frawley

Passage Press
Salt Lake City, Utah

Passage Press is a division of Morson Publishing
Morson Publishing
P.O. Box 21713
Salt Lake City, Utah 84121-0713

Published 1993

Printed in the United States of America

Cover design by Ted Nagata Graphic Design
Illustrations by Marguerite Elsbeth

Printed on acid-free paper

ISBN 1-878423-13-4

CONTENTS

Enjoyment; Rejuvenation (Rasayana);
Vajikarana, the Use of Aphrodisiacs

Part II: Methods of Ayurvedic Treatment

System (Blood or Hemoglobin Portion);
Muscular System; Adipose System; Skeletal
System; Nervous System; Reproductive
System; Urinary System; Excretory System;
Sweat System; Menstrual System; Lactation
System

EDITOR'S FOREWORD
By Dr. David Frawley

Ayurveda ("the science of life"), the traditional medicine of India, is not a science artificially imposed upon living beings. Its basis is not in dead or inorganic chemical substances, or in a mechanistic and materialistic view of the human body. Ayurveda is based upon a deep communion with the spirit of life itself and a profound understanding of the movement of the life-force and its different manifestations within our entire psycho-physical system. As such, it presents a helpful alternative to the technical and mechanical model of modern medicine, the limitations of which are gradually becoming evident through time. It is a truly holistic medicine whose wealth we have just begun to explore in the Western world.

Ayurveda is also not merely a kind of antiquated folk medicine. It is a science in its own right. Yet it is a science based upon the observation of living beings and their actual reactions to their environment. In this way, it classifies not only individuals but also foods, herbs, emotions, climates, and life-styles in an energetic language that reflects the entire living world around us.

Ayurveda possesses perhaps the longest clinical experience of any system of medicine, with a history of Ayurvedic hospitals and colleges going back for over three thousand years. It has a science of anatomy and physiology that follows a vitalistic model based upon the biological humors. It has an extensive herbal and mineral industry, including what is probably the greatest variety of herbal and pharmaceutical preparations in the world. These include herbal wines, jellies, confections, resins, balsams, pills, and an extensive system of mineral preparations. It has special clinical methods, including the use of steam therapy, oil massage, and Pancha Karma purification and rejuvenation. Perhaps most importantly, it also has a whole science of self-care, including an entire methodology of right living for optimum health and the promotion of greater awareness and creativity. All of this follows a constitutional model that considers the unique nature of the individual as the primary factor in health, not disease as an entity in itself.

While Western medicine has focused upon pathogens and how to control disease from the outside, Ayurveda concentrates on the individual and how to control disease through balancing the life-force within the individual. As the limitations of antibiotics are becoming evident, such regimes for strengthening our own internal energy or immune system may be crucial for our health as a species through the coming century. The present volume presents this science of Ayurveda in a clear and comprehensive manner. It introduces the major aspects of Ayurvedic thought and practice both for health maintenance and the treatment of disease.

The author, Dr. Subhash Ranade, is one of the most important spokespersons for Ayurveda in the world today and it is of great benefit to bring his knowledge and experience to a larger Western audience. He has been an important Ayurvedic doctor and teacher both in India and in the West for over twenty years. He has worked with many different Ayurvedic teaching programs both in India and Europe. He is the author of many books on Ayurveda including not only technical books on Ayurveda for Ayurvedic colleges but also practical books on Ayurveda and self-care for the home treatment of common diseases. This is his first book to be published in the United States. Dr. Ranade also demonstrates the wisdom of Ayurveda in his life and character, promoting the spirit as well as the form of this great tradition. It has been my pleasure to work with him over the past several years as a student, colleague, and friend and to see firsthand the scope of his understanding of health and healing.

Natural Healing Through Ayurveda provides the reader with a good idea as to the approach to Ayurveda given in Ayurvedic colleges in India today. It outlines all the essential factors of Ayurvedic study given in introductory Ayurvedic courses in India and reflects approved courses of study for foreign students. It is thorough, logical, and systematic in its approach. This allows those who are seriously interested in Ayurveda to see the full picture of its foundations. Such knowledge is necessary for all those who want to go deeper into Ayurveda at any level.

Especially useful are the sections on Ayurvedic health regimens. These outline the basic daily and seasonal practices necessary for optimal health. Also important is the long section on Yoga and Ayurveda. This shows how these two sister sciences relate together and can be used to enhance their mutual benefits. Ayurveda functions best as part of the science of Yoga and it is in light of the dissemination of Yoga to the West that Ayurveda has become known to many. Yet Ayurveda is much more detailed and specific in regard to the treatment of disease, both physical and mental, than is the system of Yoga. Hence all Yoga practitioners can benefit from some knowledge of Ayurveda.

The section on Marma points is particularly useful. Marmas, like acupuncture points, are important points on the body for redirecting energy and bringing the life-force into balance. Significant also is the section on the treatment of the channel systems. This outlines the complete scope of Ayurvedic treatment relative to all the bodily systems. The section on Pancha Karma is similarly useful in showing Ayurvedic clinical methods.

Having its foundation in Ayurvedic classics like *Charaka Samhita* and *Sushruta Samhita,* this book serves as a good introduction to these primary Ayurvedic source books. Studying it provides the reader an excellent persepective for approaching this ancient tradition.

In editing the book I have tried to remove Sanskrit terms from the main text where cumbersome for the non-specialist. Sanskrit terms have been kept in parentheses so that the reader not interested in the Sanskrit need not worry about them, while at the same time the reader who is interested can see their application. Otherwise I have added a few points here and there and have tried to make the language more understandable to the American mind. In addition I have provided in the appendix Sanskrit and herbal glossaries, which I have adapted from my own Ayurvedic Correspondence Course.

In my work of promoting the field of Vedic knowledge, I have tried not only to write books but also to edit or help publish other useful books in these areas. I feel that Dr. Ranade's work is quite valuable in this respect. We will undoubtedly see more of his many books available in the course of time.

Natural Healing Through Ayurveda will prove useful to all students of Ayurveda and to all Ayurvedic classes, courses, and study groups. It can aid in standardizing the course of study for Ayurveda in the West and establishing firm and universal principles for the teaching of Ayurveda in English. But as the science of life Ayurveda need not be adapted artificially; we must understand its principles in our own daily activities and in all aspects of our lives. Ayurveda helps us grasp the nature, meaning, and effect of our life on all levels. This is perhaps its unique gift as a medical system to humanity.

May all those who can benefit by this wisdom come to it.

Dr. David Frawley (Vamadeva Shastri)
Santa Fe, NM
January 1991

David Frawley is the author of *Ayurvedic Healing: A Comprehensive Guide; From the River of Heaven; The Astrology of the Seers; Beyond the Mind; Gods, Sages and Kings; Wisdom of the Ancient Seers;* andcoauthor of *The Yoga of Herbs.*

PREFACE

I am happy to present this work for those interested in learning the ancient healing science of Ayurveda. It was originally specially prepared for students of the C.P.A. (Certificate of Proficiency in Ayurveda) course, drafted by University of Poona in India. In order to bring uniformity to the teaching of Ayurveda for foreign students at different universities in India, Poona University arranged a National Seminar for preparing the syllabus for this course in 1984. The present book is written according to that syllabus.

I have lectured on Ayurveda in various countries since 1980, including the United States, Germany, Italy, Switzerland, and Holland. I am grateful to all the institutions who have taken the initiative to promote education in Ayurveda. In this regard, I would like to thank Mr. H. W. Schmidt of the Institute of Traditional Medicine (Saarbrucken, Ger.); Prof. Annelie Keil of the University of Bremen (Ger.); Prof Ralph Milkow of Hahnemann Collegium (Straelen, Ger.); Prof. Holger Braun and Dr. Almut Braun of Bremerhaven (Ger.); Mr. Peter Oswald of the Ashtang Yoga Akademie (Basel, Switz.); Mr. Giorgio F. Barabino of the International Association of Ayurveda and Naturopathy (Villa Era, Italy); Mrs. Lucia Mattucini of C.I.L.U.S. (Italy); Drs. Ted and Rose Ketterman of the German American Academy of Medicine (Fort Walton Beach, Fl.); Mr. Santosh Krinsky of the Institute of Wholistic Education (Wilmot, Wis.); and Mr. Steven Ross of the World Research Foundation, (Los Angeles, Cal.).

I am thankful to my wife Dr. Sunanda, who is also a graduate of Ayurveda, and has provided much help in preparing the manuscript of this book. I have received much encouragement from Mr. Anand Puranik, of Shree Dhootapapeshwar Trust, and my friends Dr. B. L. Vashta, and Dr. M. H. Paranjape. I wish to thank them all.

This book has been revised and edited by my friend, Dr. David Frawley. Dr. Frawley is a Vedic scholar and has studied Yoga, Ayurveda, and astrology in depth. He knows how to present Ayurvedic concepts to people in the United States. I am fortunate to have received his help and am quite sure that due to it this book will become more useful to readers in the West. I am very thankful to him for the service he has done to me and to Ayurveda.

After nearly two decades of work at Tilak Ayurveda College in Poona, I have recently joined Ashtang Ayurveda College and at present am working as Professor in charge of the Interdisciplinary School of Ayurvedic Medicine of Poona University. I wish to thank my friends Prof. B.V. Sathaye; Dr. M.P. Palange, principle of Ayurveda College Akurdi, Poona; Dr. B.K. Patwardhan; and other Poona University colleagues and authorities who have provided continual help in this venture.

Dr. Subhash Ranade
Rajbharati
367 Sahakar Nagar I
POONA, 4II,009 India

PART I

THE AYURVEDIC
APPROACH TO HEALTH

1
AYURVEDA
THE SCIENCE OF LIFE

He who regards kindness to humanity as the supreme religion and treats his patients accordingly, succeeds best in achieving the aims of life and obtains the greatest happiness. — *Sushruta*

Ayurveda is one of the great gifts of the sages of ancient India to mankind. It is one of the oldest scientific medical systems in the world, with a long record of clinical experience. However, it is not only a system of medicine in the conventional sense of curing disease. It is also a way of life that teaches us how to maintain and protect health. It shows us both how to cure disease and how to promote longevity. Ayurveda treats man as a "whole" — which is a combination of body, mind, and soul. Therefore it is a truly holistic and integral medical system.

The word "Ayu" means all aspects of life from birth to death. The word "Veda" means knowledge or learning. Hence Ayurveda indicates the science by which life in its totality is understood. It is a way of life that describes the diet, medicine, and behavior that are beneficial or harmful for life. The roots of Ayurveda can be traced to the beginning of cosmic creation. Indian philosophers state that Ayurveda originated from Brahma, the creator of the universe. Brahma is not a mere individual but the unmanifest form of the Divine Lord, from whom the whole manifest world comes into being. The desire to maintain fitness, health, and longevity is one of the basic instincts of all creatures. Ayurveda in this respect sets the pattern for other systems of medicine. It is a tradition with an antiquity comparable to that of life itself.

AYURVEDA AND THE VEDAS

The Vedas are regarded as the oldest and most sacred written record of knowledge.[1] The Vedas state that the Supreme Being who created the Universe, out of love and concern for humanity, gave the Divine Vedas to all mankind through the Rishis or seers of wisdom. The words of the Vedas were carefully memorized according to metrical chants and transmitted from generation to generation. Thus the four Vedas — *Rig, Yajur,*

Sama and *Atharva* — have come down to us through several thousands of years of oral transmission before finally being recorded in writing. The *Rig Veda* is the foundation stone of the other Vedas and contains, in ten books called Mandalas, 1,028 Suktas or hymns and a total of 10,572 verses. The *Yajur Veda* has 1,975 stanzas in 40 chapters of both verse and prose. The *Sama Veda* has 1,800 verses repeated from the *Rig Veda* and 75 original verses. The *Atharva Veda* has 5,977 verses, distributed among 731 Suktas.

The *Rig Veda*, the oldest of the four, contains many concepts of Ayurveda. Its three great Gods — Indra, Agni, and Soma — relate to the three biological humors of Ayurveda — Vata, Pitta, and Kapha. References are found in it to organ transplants, in the case of an artificial limb that was made for Queen Vishpala, wife of King Khela. The *Rig Veda* also contains many hymns to Soma, a Vedic God as well as a great curative herbal preparation used to treat many diseases of body and mind and to promote longevity.

Though all the Vedas contain references to Ayurvedic concepts, the *Atharva Veda* contains more of these, so much so that Ayurveda is considered to be an Upaveda or a subsidiary teaching of the *Atharva*. In the *Atharva* we find references to anatomical and physiological factors, the disease process, treatment of specific diseases, and other systematic knowledge about Ayurveda. In later ancient times, 1000–700 BC, Ayurveda developed into eight recognized branches or specialties and two prominent schools: Atreya, the School of Physicians, and Dhanvantari, the School of Surgeons.

The magico-religious aspect of medicine in the Vedas was gradually supplemented by observations based on scientific thinking. Ayurvedic scholars from subsequent generations gave a sound and logical footing of philosophy to Ayurveda. The material scattered in the Vedas was collected, subjected to rigid tests of efficacy and systematically arranged. Such compilations were called "Samhitas." Many of these compilations no longer exist. Only three authentic works have stood the test of time and are available today — the *Charaka Samhita, Sushruta Samhita,* and *Ashtanga Hridaya Samhita*. This great trio — the Brihatrayi as it is called — has enjoyed much popularity and respect for the last two thousand years. Although these texts have undergone some modification by various authors in subsequent periods, their present form is at least 1200 years old. They are all in the Sanskrit language.

CHARAKA

The *Charaka Samhita* is the oldest of the three and was probably first compiled around 1500 BC. It is considered the prime work on the basic concepts of Ayurveda.[2] Charaka represents the Atreya school of physicians. It is a systematic work divided into eight Sthanas or sections, which are further divided into 120 chapters. The first section of the *Charaka Samhita* describes the fundamental principles of Ayurveda. Then it elaborates the physiological and anatomical structure of the human body, various etiological agents, along with their role in pathogenesis, symptoms and signs of various diseases, the methodology for examination of patients, treatment, and prognosis. The preventive aspects of treatment include daily and seasonal regimens, as well as dietetics and social behavior conducive to mental health. The chapter on dietetics is a vast store of information. The section on curative treatments includes detailed descriptions of medicinal plants and their properties, various herbal preparations, and therapeutic procedures such as elimination therapy. The chapters on rejuvenation therapy and prevention of the aging process are today considered as good sources for modern research work. The *Charaka Samhita* is written in prose as well as in beautiful poetry, comparable to any Sanskrit classic. Its combined medico-social and medico-philosophical approach is a source of inspiration to anyone who studies the original text. Charaka represents the Atreya school of physicians.

SUSHRUTA

Sushruta represents the Dhanvantari school of surgeons, and is considered in Ayurveda to be the father of surgery. Even a great American society of surgeons is named after Sushruta. In the *Sushruta Samhita*[3] there are sophisticated descriptions of surgical instruments. Its classifications of fractures, wounds, abscesses, and burns as well as its elaboration of procedures for plastic surgery and anal-rectal surgery have all stood the test of time. Sushruta has also described the original concepts of pathogenesis. Sushruta describes a procedure for dissection of the human body by the maceration method. The knowledge of anatomy — bones, joints, nerves, heart, blood vessels, and circulation — is surprising and praiseworthy. The descriptions of the "marmas," vital points in the body, is comparable to the system of acupuncture points used in traditional Chinese medicine. Sushruta clearly states the importance of both theoretical and practical knowledge and describes ways and means to develop surgical skill.

THE EIGHT BRANCHES OF AYURVEDA
(ASHTANGA AYURVEDA)

1. Internal Medicine (Kayachikitsa)

Ayurveda treats man as a whole, comprising body, mind, and soul. Mind and body both affect each other and together form the seat of disease. The approach of Ayurveda from the very beginning is psychosomatic. Ayurveda groups all human beings into seven different types of constitutions (Prakriti) according to the predominance of biological humors (Doshas), and similarly groups them into seven psychological constitutions according to the predominance of mental humors. These factors are always taken into account in diagnosis, prognosis and treatment of disease. Diseases are caused by imbalance of the humors, the three energy principles, which in turn damage various tissues and systems. Pathologically, diseases have six different stages of treatment.

A number of infectious diseases are described in Ayurveda but great importance is not given to pathogens as their cause. Ayurveda emphasizes internal factors, the condition of the host, behind all diseases, even those appearing to come from the outside. It is well-known that if the soil remains sterile, the seed will not grow. In the same way, if the internal energies are balanced, disease has no field in which to act.

In the course of treatment, the Ayurvedic physician takes note of the aggravation of humors (Dosha), the tissues damaged (Dushya), environmental influences, the patient's vitality, digestive power, constitution, age, psychological factors, personal inclinations, and diet.

Ayurvedic medicines are derived from the mineral, vegetable, and animal kingdoms. More than 20,000 species of medicinal plants and herbs are found in India, out of which 2,000 are in use in Ayurveda. Six or seven hundred are commonly used in Ayurvedic preparations. A number of minerals and metals are used, but they are subject to various and complex processes of purification and oxidation before becoming suitable for internal usage. The special therapy of Pancha Karma, the five purification practices, is also used in treatment. These five are the use of emetics, purgatives, nasal medications, and medicated enemas with or without oil. Pancha Karma utilizes certain preliminary practices of Snehana (oleation internal and external) and Swedana (different kinds of fomentation or sweating therapies), and related follow-up practices like Rasayana or rejuvenation.

2. Surgery (Shalyatantra)

Surgery is not just an invention of modern medicine. It was already highly advanced in several ancient cultures, including India, Greece and Egypt. Its low condition in Europe in the Middle Ages was a period of decline, a temporary dark age, and was not at all indicative of its condition in ancient and Oriental cultures.

In Ayurveda, Sushruta describes surgery as the first and foremost specialty of the system. He describes various surgical procedures including abdominal operations like those for intestinal obstruction and stones in the bladder, and also delineates specialized surgery like plastic surgery. Sushruta was the first person to advocate knowledge of anatomy through the dissection of the dead body as essential for a good surgeon. Later in Indian history, the philosophical emphasis on non-violence came in the way of development of this branch of medicine. Even today, the *Sushruta Samhita* contains a great deal of useful material for research work. Presently efforts are being made to revive certain techniques advocated by Sushruta in the Jamnagar Institution, Benares Hindu University, and elsewhere. For example, his practice of Ksharasutra Chikitsa in ano-rectal disease has been revived. It has proved more advantageous and efficacious than modern surgical operations.

3. Shalakya Tantra

This is the Ayurvedic branch of Ophthalmology and Otorhinolaryngology, concerned with diseases of the eyes and head. Around seventy-two eye diseases are described by Sushruta along with surgical operations for such conditions as cataract and pterygium. Special techniques are also described for many diseases of the ear, nose and throat.

4. Pediatrics (Kaumarabhritya)

This branch deals with prenatal and postnatal baby care and with the care of the mother before conception and during pregnancy. Ayurveda describes methods for conceiving a child of the desired sex, intelligence, and constitution. Various diseases of children and their treatment come under this branch.

5. Toxicology (Agadatantra)

This branch deals with the toxins of the vegetable, mineral, and animal kingdoms. Most interesting to note is that the concept of pollution of air and water in particular times and places has been given due consideration. Such pollution is said to be the cause of various epidemics and the collapse of civilizations.

6. Psychiatry (Bhutavidya)

Ayurveda is equally concerned with mental diseases and their treatment. Treatment methods include not only diet and herbs, but yogic methods for improving the condition of the mind. There is ample material for further research on this branch in the *Atharva Veda* and other Ayurveda Samhitas.

7. The Science of Rejuvenation (Rasayana)

This therapy is used to prevent diseases and for promotion and prolongation of a healthy life. As mentioned earlier, Pancha Karma therapy is an essential prerequisite for Rasayana. A code of right conduct in life has also to be observed as part of the rejuvenation process. Details of regimen in terms of dietetics have also been described.

8. The Science of Aphrodisiacs (Vajikarana)

This branch deals with the means of increasing sexual vitality and efficiency. For achieving good progeny, the therapy of Rasayana and Vajikarana are closely interrelated. Vajikarana medicines also act as rejuvenatives.

The *Charaka* and *Sushruta Samhitas* prove that a vast amount of scientific research, patient investigation, and experimentation must have gone on before the conclusions recorded in them were arrived at. This period may be roughly said to be from 2000 BC to 200 BC. During this time there were great university cities in India like Takshashila, Nalanda, and Benares.

India has altitudes ranging from sea level to over twenty-five thousand feet. It has almost rainless regions and others that receive over five hundred inches a year. It has climates of extreme heat and of extreme cold. It has six clearly defined seasons, each producing its distinctive vegetation. All these climatic and geographical variations influence the body differently, along with its reaction to disease attacks and different kinds of medicines. A country with such an enormous variability of climate and such wonderful ranges of mountains as the Himalayas, the Vindhyas, and the Ghats is a rich nursery for the growth of all kinds of species of plants. It provides a vast field for botanical research. Thousands of medicinal herbs and their products, growing in diverse parts of the country in varied climates, are mentioned in Charaka and Sushruta. Diseases peculiar to different localities and seasons are also found in these books.

AYURVEDA AND BUDDHISM

The advent of Buddhism in Indian history affected all walks of life. During the period 323 BC–642 AD in which Buddhism was popular in India, the academic progress of Ayurveda was well maintained by both Hindus and Buddhists. Valuable additions were made to its literature. Most notable was a commentary on Sushruta by Nagarjuna, one of the most famous sages in the Mahayana Buddhist tradition. Yet the most remarkable thing about this period was that organized efforts were made to make the science as available as possible. Medicinal herbs were planted along the sides of public streets to be used freely by all. Many hospitals were formed. The art of nursing, which was described by Charaka, was widely practiced and systematized.

Along with Buddhist missionaries, the knowledge of Ayurveda and of Indian culture spread beyond the bounds of India. The nations of the then civilized world — including Rome, Greece, and China — were attracted toward India and students came from these countries to learn the sciences and arts of the land. The medical systems of Greece and Rome bear unmistakable signs of the influence of Ayurveda upon them. India was considered the seat of learning for the world and many philosophers and scholars visited India for study, just as many go to Europe or America today. Veterinary science was widespread in this period. Nagarjuna laid the foundation of Rasa Shastra, the use of alchemical preparations. A number of pharmaceutical preparations of Rasa medicines, special preparations of mercury, sulphur, and other minerals, and certain poisonous substances were introduced in treatment.

The medical glory of India was at its zenith during this era. In the eighth century AD, Ayurvedic physicians of India were invited to Jundishapur and Baghdad in the Middle East for consultation and were put in charge of hospitals there. During this period the culture of India spread across the oceans to the south, and across the mountains and plateaus to the north. The greater India of that day included Tibet, much of Indochina and Indonesia to the east, and extended to the west through Afghanistan and into Persia. This greater India was not built by military conquest, nor by invasions or commercial exploitation, but by devoted and humanitarian monks and yogis who carried the sacred knowledge and means of healing, both spiritual and physical.

From the second century onward we find an increasing interest in Rasakriya, pharmaceutical chemistry. During the following six centuries this study developed into a regular science (Siddha medicine) which was incorporated into Ayurveda.

VAGBHATTA

The next important authority in Ayurveda after Charaka and Sushruta is Vagbhatta of Sind, who flourished about the seventh century AD. His treatise called *Ashtanga Hridaya* presented a summary of Charaka and Sushruta with gleanings from other Ayurvedic writers like Agnivesha, Bhela, and Harita, and again brought the subject up-to-date. He introduced a number of new herbs and made valuable modifications and additions in surgery. He did all this in spite of strong opposition from the orthodox school. *Ashtanga Hridaya*[4] is classified in six sections and contains 7,444 verses in 120 chapters. The whole book is in verse.

During this time the main Ayurvedic texts were translated into Arabic. The Unani system of medicine, which the Arabs developed out of the older Greek medicine, was to a great extent founded on Ayurvedic knowledge from India. The Indian Unani system, which grew up under Muslim rule in India, never lost touch with its parental source.

The Muslim invasion of India, which began in earnest in the eleventh century and resulted in a series of wars lasting into the eighteenth century, caused a decline in Ayurveda. The violence of the conquest and its anti-Hindu and anti-Buddhist crusades weakened the older culture as a whole and made it difficult to maintain the arts and sciences at their highest level.

LATER AYURVEDIC WRITERS

Coming nearer to our times we meet with the name of Madhava or Madhavacharya, who in the twelfth century wrote several works embracing almost all branches of Hindu learning. In his medical work named *Madhava Nidana*[5] he dwells exclusively on the diagnosis of diseases. It contains 1,552 verses in 69 chapters. During the Muslim period, up to the sixteenth century, activity in Ayurveda was mainly focused on Rasakriya or alchemical preparations. Systematic works were written on the subject by Chakrapani and Vrinda. Narhari Pandita and Madanpal wrote two masterpieces on medicinal herbs, *Raja Nighantu* and *Madanpala Nighantu*. Sharangdhara, the son of Damodara, in the fourteenth century systematized various materia medicas and his is still a most popular and reliable treatise on the subject. His book contains 2,500 verses, is divided into three parts and has 32 chapters. The *Sharangdhara Samhita*[6], *Madhava Nidana,* and *Bhava Prakasha* are regarded as the Laghu Traya or Junior Triad of Ayurvedic classics.

The next celebrated writer on Ayurveda is Bhavamishra, the author of *Bhava Prakasha*[7]. This physician lived in the sixteenth century and was considered to be the best scholar of his time in northwest India. His treatise contains 10,831 verses and is divided into three sections. Its style is simple and delightful to read. In the time of Bhavamishra, India began to come into contact with the European nations, notably the Portuguese, who were attracted by trade. A syphilitic disease, in which hands and feet were affected, was then common among the Portuguese. Bhavamishra deals with this[8] at length under the name of Firanga Roga, Foreigner's disease.

BRITISH INFLUENCE ON AYURVEDA
AND MODERN TIMES

The advent of the British was another big landmark in the decline of Ayurveda. The British not only denied state patronage to Ayurveda, they also took a negative attitude toward the system. The East India Company closed down existing schools of Ayurveda and started a medical school of their own at Calcutta in 1833. In spite of suppression and the lack of patronage, Ayurveda remained popular with the masses and still served about 80% of the population of the country. The tremendous national awakening around 1920, with the establishment of national schools and universities, encouraged the revival of Ayurveda. Different state governments were compelled to start regular teaching of Ayurveda and thus established state boards, faculties and councils of Indian medicine.

The government of India also appointed a committee under the chairmanship of Sir R. N. Chopra in 1946, which made several recommendations for teaching and research in Ayurveda.

After independence, the government of India and the state governments took more interest in Ayurveda. Over fifty universities in India now have faculties of Ayurveda and over one-hundred Ayurvedic colleges are affiliated with these universities.

Presently the government of India has initiated a more open policy and allows the founding of more private Ayurvedic institutions on a non-grant basis. Therefore many new Ayurvedic schools are arising all over India today. In the next decade the scope of Ayurvedic education in India should expand greatly. Ayurveda in the twenty-first century looks to inherit its old glory of ancient times and will be one of the most important forms of naturopathic medicine practiced in the world.

In this event it is especially important for the presentation of Ayurveda to be updated so that it may best continue to stand the test of time. It should be studied rationally using modern experimental methods from various disciplines of science and technology. This does not mean Ayurveda should accommodate itself to allopathic medicine and its standards, which are not appropriate for it, but that it has to be presented in a clear, modern and rational language, and subject itself to proof through observation and clinical experience.

AYURVEDA AND THE PHILOSOPHIES OF INDIA

Ayurveda is not only a science, it is a philosophy as well. All Indian sciences have a basis in philosophy. Such philosophies are not merely logical systems but reflect profound meditative experience. Ayurveda, which deals with the maintenance, improvement and prolongation of life in general and human life in particular, observes nature and the universe for its attributes and actions. Ayurveda accepts the Vedic view that the Microcosm (individual) and Macrocosm (universe) are identical and that Man is the miniature of Nature. Hence Ayurveda is concerned with theories of evolution and the creation of the universe.

The various philosophies of India deal with the process of creation from different points of view. Six systems of philosophy derive from the Vedas and are called Vedic systems. Those which do not base themselves upon the Vedas are called non-Vedic systems. The main contribution to Ayurveda has come through the Vedic systems, of which Sankhya-Yoga and Nyaya-Vaisheshika are the most important.

NYAYA-VAISHESHIKA

The Nyaya system deals with the means of knowledge or proofs (Pramanas). It accepts four such means of right knowledge: Pratyaksha or direct perception via the senses and mind, Anumana or inference, Upamana or analogy, and Shabda or the word spoken by an authority. Ayurveda in principle accepts these four means for arriving at the truth of things.

The Vaisheshika system deals with the creation of the universe and explains six categories of knowledge or objects of cognition (Prameyas). These are substance (dravya), quality (guna), action (karma), similarity (samanya), dissimilarity (vishesha), and unbreakable relation (samavaya).

Vaisheshika presents an atomic theory of creation (Paramanuvada). According to it, the earth, water, light (fire), and the principle of motion (air) are created by combining the atoms of these basic substances. The mind also has a single atom in every individual. Ayurveda similarly states that the body is developed by the union of various body particles.

According to Vaisheshika, the diversity observable in the universe comes from the transformation of the atoms of earth (gross matter) resulting from their contact with heat. Ayurveda accepts this theory and states that all the transformations in the body, both anabolic and catabolic, only occur due to the existence of the fire principle (Agni) in the body. If this heat principle is normal, health is maintained, and if it is abnormal, disease is produced. Death occurs when Agni ceases to function in the body.

Similar substances, qualities and actions are responsible for increase in the bodily substances of the three biological humors (Doshas), seven tissues (Dhatus), and three waste-materials (Malas). This is the simple principle of like increases like. Antagonistic substances, qualities, and actions decrease these same factors. This is the principle that things are balanced or cured by their opposites. For maintaining health and curing disease, one has to understand these similarities and antagonisms according to the causative factors of health and disease.

Bodily substances are increased by the utilization and assimilation of similar substances taken from the outside world and are decreased by the use of antagonistic substances. Hence the Ayurvedic principle of treatment in health and in disease (i.e. diet and behavior) is to use either similar or antagonistic means according to the requirements of the particular condition.

Ayurvedic pharmaceutical theory is based upon the description given in Vaisheshika of dravya, guna, and karma. Substances (dravya) create actions (karma) according to their qualities (guna). Hot substances produce heat while cold substances produce cold. Ayurveda describes twenty qualities of the five basic substances called the five great elements. All substances are applied accoding to the principle of similarity and antagonism.

SANKHYA AND YOGA

Though Ayurveda utilizes certain important principles of Vaisheshika, the Sankhya and Yoga system provides the basic philosophy for Ayurveda. The Sankhya theory of creation does not stop at the level of five elements like that of Vaisheshika, but stresses the ultimate cause at the most subtle level. Though there are five categories of knowledge at the level of the sense organs, there are three at the level of mind and only one at the level of the intellect. Every sensation can be analyzed at a mental level into three types — pleasurable, neutral, or painful. They are explained by Sankhya as the three gunas — Sattva, Rajas, and Tamas. The combined or balanced form of these three gunas is called Prakriti or primal Nature, which is the ultimate cause of this creation.

The process of knowing occurs at the level of the intellect only, irrespective of the pleasurable, painful, or neutral nature of the knowledge. Therefore, there must be some other ultimate principle which is responsible for this knowing and it must be ever knowing. Sankhya calls this principle Purusha or pure consciousness.

Prakriti and its three gunas are responsible for the diversity in the universe, while the existence of the Purusha is responsible for unity. These two, Prakriti and Purusha, are the ultimate, causeless, omnipresent, and all pervasive causes of the universe. When they combine, creation starts and when they get detached, creation comes to an end. The ending of creation according to Sankhya is the merging of creation back into its creator or the effect back into cause.

The soul in living beings reflects the Purusha, while the material vestures — including body, mind and intellect — derive from Prakriti. The aim of Sankhya is to give detachment and liberation (moksha) to the Purusha. The permanent detached state of the soul is the absolute state of joy which is everlasting. Most of the philosophies of India have this state of liberation as their ultimate goal.

Though Ayurveda accepts the absolute detachment of the soul and describes the highest goal of treatment as the state of liberation, for practical purposes it does not emphasize it. It does not advise the neglect of the body, though it is perishable, but stresses the need to care for it, prevent its premature destruction, promote its stability, and infuse it with vitality and vigor in order to prolong its existence. At the same time, it also advises one to exercise self-restraint, to cultivate detachment, and to make efforts for self-realization. The Purusha (soul) associated with Prakriti (the body) is considered by Ayurveda as the real individual for the practical purposes of promoting health and curing disease. Hence Ayurveda addresses the needs of the ordinary person.

From these two basic principles, Prakriti and Purusha, Sankhya outlines the twenty-three basic principles of existence, shown in the following table —

Purusha, Pure Consciousness
Prakriti, Great Nature
Cosmic Intelligence (Mahat)
Cosmic Ego (Ahankara)

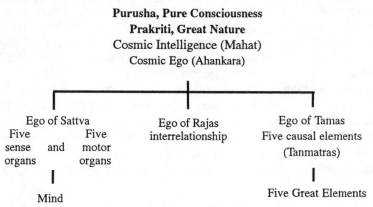

Ego of Sattva		Ego of Rajas	Ego of Tamas
Five sense organs	and Five motor organs	interrelationship	Five causal elements (Tanmatras)
Mind			Five Great Elements

The Ayurvedic view of creation is very practical. It assumes the creation of the organs of sense and action from the five gross elements only. (Sankhya considers their origin to be from the Tamasic ego.) Sankhya considers the Purusha as a completely separate entity from Prakriti, while Ayurveda accepts the soul which is united with the body or Prakriti.

Sankhya states that according to the law of transformation (Parinamavada) Prakriti, as a composition of the three gunas, is always in a state of flux. Due to the endless combinations of these three basic qualities, changes occur at every moment. Ayurveda accepts this law of transformation and explains it as the reason for creation and destruction, occurring both in the body and the world.

At the level of the sense organs and mind, increase in Sattva, the quality of purity, gives right knowledge to the intellect, provides courage and determination to avoid harmful but momentarily pleasant things and gives an alert memory. Hence, increase in Sattva by the regulation of diet and behavior is recommended by Ayurveda. On the other hand, an increase in either Rajas or Tamas, the qualities of agitation and dullness in the mind, is responsible for wrong decisions, fearfulness, and loss of memory.

The Yoga system aids Ayurveda by providing methods for increasing Sattva, decreasing Rajas and Tamas, and thereby balancing the mind. To achieve this, Yoga gives a regimen of diet and behavior, called Yama and Niyama.

MIMAMSA AND VEDANTA

These two philosophies have also contributed to Ayurveda. Mimamsa says that every soul or Purusha is everlasting and travels through the great cycle of birth and death. One experiences pain or pleasure according to the deeds performed in this or previous lives. The incurability of certain diseases is explained in Ayurveda by this law of karma. Not all diseases are amenable to physical or even psychological treatment. Some diseases occur owing to karma and must be experienced, or can only be alleviated by spiritual or religious purification methods.

The Ayurvedic view of the inherent freedom of the Soul (Atman) from all bonds of pain and pleasure and the ultimate union of the individual soul with the universal soul is taken from Vedanta. Ayurveda, like Vedanta, is based upon the principle of self-knowledge and aims at self-realization, the knowledge of the One or Divine Self in all beings. Also, according to Vedanta each of the gross elements develops by the combination of all the five primordial elements (Tanmatras). Departing from Sankhya, Ayurveda accepts this concept of Vedanta.

NON-VEDIC PHILOSOPHIES

Ayurveda is based primarily on Vedic philosophies. Yet it can also be found useful from the standpoint of Buddhist, Jain and other non-Vedic philosophies, from which it has borrowed some points. Jain thinkers state the law of uncertainty or all probabilities (Naikantavada), that any number of points of view on any subject are always possible. From the standpoint of diagnosis and treatment, Ayurveda accepts this law of probabilities. One cannot definitely know all such factors and hence one's approach should always be capable of modification.

The Buddha teaches that creation is a momentary affair; that each thing gets destroyed in the next moment (Kshanabhangavada). Ayurveda uses this law as a part of treatment by the avoidance of causative factors. Pathology gets destroyed of its own and health gets re-established when the causative factors that produce it disappear. Ayurvedic treatment seeks to remove the cause of disease and health will return of its own accord.

Since all the important Indian philosophies have contributed to the development of Ayurveda, the study of their essential principles is helpful for all students of Ayurveda. Ayurveda finds many different philosophies useful to it. It has a place for most of the philosophies of the world within its system, as its aim is the maximum integration of human knowledge toward the maximum fulfillment of life.

2
FUNDAMENTAL
PRINCIPLES OF AYURVEDA

There is no end to the learning of Ayurveda. Hence you should carefully and constantly devote yourself to it. You should increase your skill by learning from others without jealousy. The wise regard the whole world as their teacher, whereas the ignorant consider it to be their enemy.

— *Charaka*

Ayurveda is the science of positive health and fulfillment in life. The aim of Ayurveda is threefold:

- To achieve positive health for the individual
- Protection of the masses
- Ultimate liberation

The last goal can be achieved by following regulations of daily conduct and by following strict seasonal regimens, so that one can be constantly healthy. Being continuously healthy is comparable to achieving ultimate liberation, as it involves the eradication of the factors that bring about suffering.

The entire approach of Ayurveda is based upon the basic urge in the body for protection of life. From the beginning of life there is the instinct to protect it from negative effects. Universally pervasive substances, like the five great elements, do not change their properties. The moon and water act as cooling agents, while the sun acts as an agent for thermal heat. The properties of such substances are demonstrated naturally. Proof by laboratory techniques is not required. For example, we do not need an experiment to show that fire burns; its burning quality is inseparable from its nature.

The drugs employed in modern medical sciences have been changing rapidly, while the basic nature of the human body has remained the same. When drugs used for a period of time become ineffective it indicates that something is fundamentally wrong with our entire approach to healing.

As against this, the principles and methods of Ayurveda have remained constant since its inception.

Ayurveda accepts the concept of a common origin for the universe and man. The universe is the macrocosm, while man is the microcosm. For the creation of the universe, two types of substances are essential — material and immaterial. There must be both material form and an immaterial essence underlying its variations and combinations. Both of these are also present in man.

THE THREE GUNAS OR PRIMARY QUALITIES

Consciousness or intelligence (Sattva), motion or action (Rajas), and the inertia which resists them (Tamas) are called the "three gunas" (trigunas). They are the three primary and omnipresent qualities at work behind all material forms in nature. For the creation of any substance in the universe, the contribution of these three non-material consituents is essential.

Ideological conception (Sattva), material reorganization (Rajas), and inhibition for both (Tamas) are the three real factors behind the apparent existence of any substance. These three primary qualities by themselves do not have any form, hence they are called non-material substances. These three gunas are also manifest in human beings in the the qualities of their temperament, constitution and behavior.

THE FIVE GREAT ELEMENTS

The basic material constituents which exist in the universe and in man are called the "five great elements" (Pancha Mahabhutas) of ether, air, fire, water, and earth. The original substance of this group pervades the universe and is not completely observable, hence it is called the "great element" (Mahabhuta). These elements refer to the etheric, gaseous, radiant, fluid, and solid states of matter and their respective principles of space, movement, light, cohesion, and density. Hence they are far more subtle and comprehensive than their visible counterparts on earth. According to the Sankhya-Yoga system they evolve from the mind.

Each of these primal elements possesses its characteristic quality (either essential or auxiliary). The essential qualities of sound (ether), touch (air), light and color (fire), taste (water), and smell (earth) are grasped by the corresponding five sense organs of the ear, skin, eye, tongue, and nose. When these are not perceived, the alternative five auxiliary characteristics are observed indirectly through the skin. They are non-resistance (ether), vibrations (air), change of temperature (fire), fluidity (water), and shape (earth).

CHARACTERISTICS OF THE FIVE ELEMENTS

Elements	Essential	Auxiliary	Related to
Ether AKASHA	Sound	Non-resistance	Rarefaction
Air VAYU	Touch	Vibration	Propulsion
Fire TEJAS	Appearance	Heat & Color	Conversion
Water APAS	Taste	Fluidity	Degree of Liquidity
Earth PRITHIVI	Smell	Solidity	Density of Particles

TRIDOSHA THEORY: THE THREE BIOLOGICAL HUMORS

The scientists of old explained all body functions relative to the happenings in the universe. They found certain phenomena common to both man and nature. There are three main causative factors in the external universe: the sun, moon and wind. The sun is the energy of conversion represented as fire. The moon is the agency of cooling represented by the combination of earth and water. The wind is the principle of movement or propulsion represented by the combination of air and ether.

All activities in the universe or in the human being are grouped into the three basic functions of creation, preservation, and destruction. These are the functions of three main Hindu Gods of Brahma, Vishnu, and Shiva. The Tridosha theory relates these three functions to the three biological humors or Doshas. Vata, the energetic humor, controls destruction. Pitta, the thermogenic humor, organizes body activities after transformation. Kapha, the cohesive humor, is responsible for maintaining the creation.

RELATION OF THE FIVE ELEMENTS
TO THE THREE ENERGY PRINCIPLES IN THE UNIVERSE

STRUCTURE OF UNIVERSE			FUNCTIONS IN UNIVERSE
Ether	Space		Principle of
		WIND	propulsion, movement
Air	Motion		
Fire	Energy	SUN	Principle of conversion, transformation
Water	Cohesion		Principle of cooling,
		MOON	cohesion or preservation
Earth	Mass		

UNIVERSEL FUNCTION	MAN
Principle of propulsion	Vata Dosha
Principle of conversion	Pitta Dosha
Principle of preservation	Kapha Dosha

RELATIONSHIP OF FIVE ELEMENTS, THREE GUNAS, & TRIDOSHA

Elements	Gunas	Humors	Gunas
Ether	Sattva		
		VATA	Sattva 1 + Rajas 1
Air	Rajas		
Fire	Sattva + Rajas	PITTA	Sattva 1 + Rajas 1
Water	Sattva + Tamas		
		KAPHA	Sattva 1 + Tamas 2
Earth	Tamas		

All the natural happenings observable in the universe are caused by one of the three energies:

- Agency of propulsion
- Agency of interchanging
- Agency of cohesion

This energy of propulsion causes the change in position of all things in the universe — like dust, smoke and clouds — in the direction in which the wind or force of propulsion is moving. In human beings, functions like respiration, heart beat, and the expulsion of waste products all are manifestations of change in position.

The energy inside the body is termed Vata, which is similar to wind (Vata itself also means wind). But it must be remembered that Vata should not be simply equated with wind. This is an analogy. Vata is any propulsive force and the principle of movement generally on the level of the life-force (Prana). The lower part of the large intestine is the seat of this humor. The functions manifested here (drying of the waste matter by removing the liquid portion) resemble those of the wind in nature.

When any substance comes in contact with the heat of the sun, it changes its temperature, form, appearance, or taste. In the human body the same type of thermogenic energy causes the food taken in to be changed into tissues and waste products. It is responsible for the complexion and temperature of the body. Hence it is named Pitta, that which is thermogenic in nature. Sweat, which is increased by heat, and blood, which is red in color, thus having properties common to fire, are the main seats of Pitta.

The effects of these two energies are inhibited by the third energy, the agency of cold and cohesion or, in nature, the rainfall. This is responsible for new growth. Hence it is named Kapha, or that which gets activated by water. The nutrient fluid pool, secretions, muscular tissues, bony structures, the nervous system, and the reproductive system are the chief sites of this humor.

HUMORS, TISSUES, AND WASTE MATERIALS: DOSHA, DHATU, AND MALA

Ayurvedic scientists have classified all bodily constituents into three categories. They are Dosha, Dhatu, and Mala — the humors, tissues, and waste materials.

Mala or the waste products are the constituents that are constantly eliminated from the body. Their physical appearance varies from gaseous, liquid, semi-solid to solid form. The gross waste products (sthula) are urine, feces, and sweat. The subtle waste products (sukshma malas or kleda) are exudations eliminated from the epithelial linings of the eyes, nose, mouth, ears, and smegma. Similarly, the many minute waste products that are formed in the body during tissue formation from food are also included in subtle waste materials. Health is maintained when these waste products are eliminated properly. When they accumulate in excess, various diseases are produced.

Dhatus or tissues are the constituents which do not get eliminated from the body (except the reproductive) and they are maintained within a particular limit. This limit is the skin from the outside and the internal linings (of the gastro-intestinal tract, bladder, joints, and cerebral linings) from within the body. As bodily strength grows these tissues continue to develop. They are seven in number, with their characters and functions as follows:

NAME	CHARACTER	FUNCTION
Rasa Dhatu PLASMA	Circulating nutrient fluid	Nutrition
Rakta Dhatu BLOOD	Hemoglobin portion of the blood	Oxygenation
Mamsa Dhatu MUSCLE	Muscular tissue	Movement
Meda Dhatu FAT	Lubricating fat deposits	Lubrication

Asthi Dhatu BONE	Supporting and accommodating bony structures	Support
Majja Dhatu NERVE	Nerve tissues	To promote understanding
Shukra Dhatu REPRODUCTIVE	Reproductive tissue	Reproduction

The most important function of this group is to give maximum support and strength to the body. The body cannot afford to eliminate the tissues in this group like the waste materials. If they cross the limit of the skin or the internal linings, then the disease condition becomes very serious, as essential substances are being lost.

The humors (Doshas) play a dual role. They do not continue developing like the tissues, nor are they completely eliminated from the body like the waste materials. Vata has no physical form. It is understood by the various movements it sets in motion. Pitta and Kapha are of a fluid character, Pitta consisting of lighter fluids and Kapha of heavier fluids.

Formation of Vata

The movements of breathing and swallowing trigger the cycle leading to absorption of external food. This movement also depends upon previously absorbed food. Thus Indian scientists have understood a relationship between energy and food absorption. Hence Vata is described as the ejectable product of food. Anna Mala, the waste material from food = Vata Dosha. This energy is then utilized by the body for essential movements like breathing, heart beat, passage of food, excretion of waste products, and so on. These movements cannot be measured or weighed. Thus Vata is perceived by the totality of its functions.

Formation of Pitta and Kapha

The movements that appear in the upper part of the gastro-intestinal tract disappear during the process of absorption of food. Saliva and mucous secretions (Kapha) and other digestive secretions including various enzymes and hormones (Pitta) appear in the proximal part and then re-enter in the distal part with absorbed food.

Kapha, when it appears in the mouth, gastro-intestinal tract, lungs, or cerebral circulation is the ejectable product from Rasa Dhatu, the plasma or the nutrient body fluid. Such Kapha Dosha looses certain characteristics of Rasa Dhatu. Hence Rasa Mala, the waste product of the Rasa or plasma, = Kapha.

When it leaves the circulating channels this nutrient fluid forms various tissues according to need: it may change into muscle tissue, provide its lubricating material for adipose tissue, or help in the formation of bones, nerves, or reproductive fluids. The channeled nutrient fluid is Kapha Dosha because it helps in the cohesion of various tissues.

Pitta is the product of the breakdown of the blood (Rakta Dhatu). Rakta Mala, the waste product of the blood = Pitta Dosha. This Pitta Dosha appears as colored secretions in the middle portion of the gastro-intestinal tract and is thus responsible for the central conversion function. The blood (Rakta) does not combine with any other constituent in the body. Hence it is different from other tissues. Pitta Dosha, however, which is a breakdown product of hemoglobin, helps in various conversions; in the eye for vision, in the skin for complexion, and in the liver for formation of various tissues.

PROPERTIES OF THE THREE HUMORS

Vata is recognized by its qualities as dry, cool, rough, less nourishing, propulsive, and subtle. It possesses an astringent taste. When the living body comes into contact with substances of such qualities, it loses bodily constituents. Even though these qualities are harmful to existing tissues in the body, they are essential for body functions. If subtleness in the structure of a tissue is nullified, there can be no movement in it at all.

Pitta is slightly oily in character, has a sharp odor, secretory and vasodilating properties, is penetrating and hot, and is pungent and sour in taste. In the process of digestion it appears as an easily flowing fluid. All colors except white, dusky or violet denote the existence of Pitta.

Kapha is oily, cool, smooth, soft, heavy, nourishing, slimy, compact in arrangement, white in color, and is sweet and salty by taste.

Functions of Vata

As the principle of propulsion, Vata carries out many diverse functions in the human body. It controls cell arrangement and division, the formation of different tissue layers, and the differentiation of organs and systems. It conducts impulses like those from the sense organs to the brain and from the brain to the motor organs. Vata controls the expulsion of feces, urine, sweat, menstrual fluid, semen, and the fetus. It also controls respiratory, cardiac and gastro-intestinal movements, as well as all higher functions in the brain and spinal cord. Vata controls the mind and gives the energy to perform all bodily and mental activities.

Functions of Pitta

Pitta is responsible for the formation of tissues, waste products, and energy from the food, water, and air that we take in from the outside. It controls metabolic activities and is responsible for all the secretions in the gastro-intestinal tract, and the enzymes and hormones from ductless glands into the blood stream. It controls body temperature, hunger, thirst, fear, anxiety, anger, and sexual desire. Pitta is also responsible for courage and will power, and assimilation of knowledge from the outside world.

Functions of Kapha

Kapha increases the deposits in the cell mass as well as being essential for the interlinking of cells, tissues, and organs. It is thus responsible for the growth of the body. It prevents destruction of tissues from wear and tear — due to friction and movement by Vata — by maintaining the strength and immunity of the body. Capacities for reproduction, happiness, and correct retention of knowledge depend upon the proper functioning of Kapha.

Ayurveda attributes great importance to the equilibrium of the three humors or Tridosha. Although they are in a constant state of flux, due to the impact of internal and external factors, their equilibrium is usually maintained. When this equilibrium gets disturbed, the disease process starts. According to the Indian system of medicine, all diseases are caused by aggravated humors or vitiated Doshas. Even traumatic diseases which are not initially the result of an imbalance of these Doshas soon become accompanied by one.

TYPES OF THE HUMORS

According to different functions and sites, each humor is divided into five types.

TYPES OF VATA

The five types of Vata are Prana, Udana, Vyana, Samana, and Apana. All these forms of Vata are responsible for various propulsive movements.

Prana — Udana

These two, having opposite movements, are taken together. Generally speaking the movement of Prana is from the outside to the inside. Prana is responsible for receiving substances like air, water, food, and impressions through the five sense organs from the outside world. Whenever a sound, touch, taste, or smell is attended with full concentration, it has some effect on respiration.

The movement of Udana is from the inside to the outside, mainly through exhalation. Substances received by the stomach in fluid (like alcohol) or solid form (like garlic), if rendered very fine during the conversion of food, are eliminated through expiration. Speech is also due to Udana. Remembrance is the bringing out of the knowledge that has been received by Prana. Thus Prana is responsible for intake, Udana for output.

Vyana — Samana

These two types of Vata also have opposite propulsion. Vyana is responsible for propulsion from center to periphery. The movement of the heart in pushing nutritive substances to the periphery is the function of Vyana. It is also responsible for various movements of the limbs and the flow of blood and sweat. Vyana carries afferent impulses from the sense organs to the brain.

Samana, on the other hand, is the propulsive force from the periphery to the center. Efferent impulses in the nerves, bringing all the fluid pushed out by Vyana back to the center and promoting all fluids into the lumen, are the function of Samana. Thus the action of Samana is the central pull action opposite the outward push of Vyana.

Apana

In contrast to the above two pairs, the function of Apana is to control the movements of constituents like urine, feces, flatus, menstrual discharge, seminal discharge, and the discharge of the fetus. All these are controlled for a particular period of time before being discharged from the body. The overall control of all these substances for a particular period is beneficial to building or maintaining the tissues. Since this control is beneficial to the other types of Vata, it is said that Apana controls all the different forms of Vata.

TYPES OF PITTA

The five types of Pitta are Pachaka, Ranjaka, Alochaka, Sadhaka, and Bhrajaka. All of these are responsible for some type of conversion.

Pachaka Pitta

Pachaka Pitta is responsible for the primary conversion in the body, the digestion of food. Because of its hot and penetrating quality it disintegrates and digests food in the gastro-intestinal tract.

Ranjaka Pitta

Ranjaka Pitta aids in the secondary digestion of food for the formation of tissues. The formation of blood (Rakta) and other tissues in the liver is the chief function of Ranjaka Pitta.

Alochaka Pitta

Alochaka Pitta is responsible for the assimilation and conversion of external impulses that takes place when an object is sensed by the eyes. It is inferred that the sensations of sound, touch, taste, and smell also involve a certain conversion. The factor responsible for this conversion is Alochaka Pitta.

Sadhaka Pitta

Sadhaka Pitta is located in the brain. After sensing any object, its recognition is dependent upon a specific sequence of conversions governed by Sadhaka Pitta. The capacity to appreciate art is another function of it.

Bhrajaka Pitta

Bhrajaka Pitta maintains the temperature and complexion of the skin, and helps in the absorption of massage oils and ointments through the skin.

TYPES OF KAPHA

The five types of Kapha are Avalambaka, Kledaka, Bodhaka, Tarpaka, and Shleshaka. All of these protect various organs from wear and tear due to Vata and the hot and penetrating effects of Pitta. Similarly they help maintain the cohesion and interlinking of tissues.

Avalambaka Kapha

Avalambaka Kapha protects the lungs, heart, and proximal portion of the intestines. Due to repeated contraction and relaxation, the lungs and heart are subjected to friction and wear. But the fine, slimy and unctuous secretions inside these organs protect them and preserve their integrity.

Kledaka Kapha

Kledaka Kapha protects the upper and middle abdomen from hot, irritant or cold food as well as from the secretions of Pachaka Pitta.

Bodhaka Kapha

Bodhaka Kapha protects the mouth from pungent, hot, cold or irritating food and drinks. It also helps us to taste food. Potentially harmful substances are initially rejected by this taste screen.

Shleshaka Kapha

Shleshaka Kapha lubricates all the bony ends of the joints and prevents their friction during movements.

Tarpaka Kapha

Tarpaka Kapha provides various nutrients to the brain cells and gives lubrication and protection to the brain and spinal cord.

✳ ✳ ✳

DIGESTION OF FOOD
The Role of Agni, the Digestive Fire

The agency of conversion in the universe is represented in the physical body by the power of Agni, which literally means "fire." It refers to the principle of transformation in all its potencies and appearances, which we most commonly experience in the outer world of nature in the form of fire. Such a principle of conversion appears throughout the universe in the various changes of substances such as those observed in biochemical, chemical, and nuclear processes. It serves to transform the gross into the subtle, in which process energy is released and new forms are created. In the body, Agni serves to convert food into various body constituents. This conversion takes place by three types of Agni working at three different levels.

The Digestive Fire (Jatharagni)

The Digestive Fire is the agency responsible for digesting food in the small intestine. It is also called "Kayagni," the bodily fire, as it is the main source of heat in the body. This energy converts food into a uniform suspension or homogeneous mass (Ahara Rasa).

Digestive Power in the Tissues (Dhatvagni)

Dhatvagni is essential for the second stage of conversion. Dhatvagnis are the special digestive agencies for the various bodily tissues (Dhatus). For the formation of each tissue a separate Dhatvagni is required. Thus there are seven Dhatvagnis for the seven tissues. Dhatvagni is dependent on Jatharagni. If the activity of the Dhatvagni is too low or too high it results in the malformation of the particular tissue. If the tissue Agni is too high, the tissue gets burnt up or depleted. If it is too low, an excess of low quality tissue is formed.

Power of Digestion on an Elemental Level (Bhutagni)

Bhutagni is required for the third stage of digestion, the formation of special materials for the sense organs. There are five Bhutagnis for taking the five element portions of the digested food mass (Ahara Rasa) and converting them into nutritive substances for the five sense organs. Some of these specialized materials are the rods and cones responsible for photosensitivity in the eye, special liquids around the taste buds on the tongue, mucous membrane material inside the nose, and the substances forming the architecture of the ear. Such substances specific to each sense organ (Indriya Dravya) are prepared by the Bhutagnis.

PROCESS OF DIGESTION

The process of digestion has two components, namely the primary phase of digestion (Avasthapaka), and post-digestive effect (Vipaka).

The Primary Phase of Digestion (Avasthapaka)

This is also divided into three stages named according to the prevalence of tastes (rasas) operative during them.

The sweet stage of digestion (Madhura Avasthapaka) is the stage of liquefaction. During this stage Kledaka Kapha secretions occur in the stomach and the disintegration of the food takes place. Due to the heavy secretionary action of Kledaka Kapha, there is a reduction of activity in the body after eating.

The sour digestive stage (Amla Avasthapaka) is the stage of acidification. Secretion of Pachaka Pitta, digestive juices and enzymes, which occurs mainly in the small intestine, breaks down the food further. It causes a sensation of thirst and perspiration through its creation of heat.

The pungent digestive stage (Katu Avasthapaka) is the stage of alkalization of food. About four and a half hours after eating, the food passes into the distal part of the gastrointestinal tract, the large intestine, and peristaltic movements are diminished. During this stage there arises a desire to move about in contrast to the first phase of digestion. This stage is due to the transient predominance of Vata.

Post-Digestive Effect (Vipaka)

The post-absorption action of food is also described in three categories. But it must be remembered that primary (Avasthapaka) stages occur for every food type. The post-digestive effect can be either sweet

(Madhura Vipaka), sour (Amla Vipaka), or pungent (Katu Vipaka), depending upon the quality of the food.

If sweet post-digestive effect (Madhura Vipaka) is formed, the body receives nutrition of all types and excretory products are easily discharged. Sour post-digestive effect (Amla Vipaka) indicates that the body will be poorly nourished but the waste products will be eliminated smoothly. Pungent post-digestive effect (Katu Vipaka) means that the body will neither receive proper nutrition nor it will easily eliminate waste products. Thus the post-digestive effect denotes the ultimate result of the process of digestion in the body.

✳ ✳ ✳

MOVEMENT OF THE DOSHAS THROUGH THE CYCLE OF TIME

	KAPHA	PITTA	VATA
DAY	7 am–11 am	11 am–3 pm	3 pm–7 pm
NIGHT	7 pm–11 pm	11 pm–3 am	3 am–7 am
SEASON	Feb. 7– Jun. 7	June 7–Oct.7	Oct. 7–Feb. 7
DIGESTION	1st 1 ½ hour	2nd 1 ½ hour	3rd 1 ½ hour

The Doshas also reflect the rhythms of time. They show how the forces of nature discharge their effects according to the changes of time periods and developments of various processes of transformation.

In the cycle of the day, Kapha is dominant in the morning and evening; Pitta predominates at noon and midnight; Vata is highest at sunrise and sunset, the transitional points of the day. Seasonally, Kapha is highest in late winter and early spring, the seasons of cold and dampness; Pitta is highest in the late spring and summer, the seasons of heat; Vata is highest in the fall and early winter, the seasons of cold and dryness.

In the digestive process, Kapha is highest immediately after eating. Hence nausea right after food intake indicates high Kapha. Pitta is highest two or three hours after eating, at which time it may be experienced as heartburn. Vata is highest at the end of the digestive process, evidenced as symptoms like gas or constipation. It is best to treat the Doshas at their respective times. Hence medicines to decrease Kapha are given in the morning, for Pitta in the afternoon, and for Vata in the evening.

3
INDIVIDUAL CONSTITUTION:
PRAKRITI

Ayurvedic treatment is based upon the ascertainment of individual constitution. This is the unique power of the system in that it treats the living individual as the most important factor. Ayurveda does not regard disease as a factor in itself but only as a complication of constitutional imbalance. Hence it regards disease more as a product of how we live than as an attack from the outside.

The predominance of elements, gunas and Doshas at the time of fertilization decides the constitution or bio-typology of the individual. Once this proportion is set it generally remains permanent for the lifetime of the individual. The Prakriti or physical constitution of an individual depends upon the following:

- Condition of sperm and ovum at the time of conception

- Nature of the season and the condition inside the uterus

- Food & other regimens adopted by mother during pregnancy

- Nature of the elements comprising the fetus

The physical constitution is also influenced by class, family traits, locality, time, age, and individuality. The predominance of elements decides the physical constitution, while the predominance of gunas decides the psychological constitution. The predominance of humors (Doshas) determines the functional or Doshic Prakriti, the energetic condition of the body. Of these types of constitution, the classification of humoral dominance is most important in the examination of both health and disease. Hence the Doshic Prakriti is the focus of Ayurveda.

FUNCTIONAL OR DOSHIC CONSTITUTION

Based on the permutations and combinations of the three Doshas, seven types of constitutions can be formed:

- Vata
- Kapha
- Vata-Kapha
- Pitta
- Vata-Pitta
- Pitta-Kapha
- Sannipata or balanced constitution (Sama Prakriti)

These types are classified by their predominance. We find that a purely single Dosha constitution is seldom found and although a balanced constitution is extremely good, this type is also rare.

Vata constitution is usually inferior in terms of health and longevity; Pitta is usually in between; and Kapha is usually superior. Of the dual constitutions, Pitta-Kapha type is difficult for health and longevity; Vata-Kapha type more difficult; and Vata-Pitta most difficult. Sama Prakriti, or the constitution in which all three Doshas are in equal proportion, is best. The important characteristics of each constitution are described in the chart included in this chapter. In addition, we present below a brief sketch of each of the three main types.

Vata Constitution

These people usually have tall or thin bodily frames and less strength. Their body weight is low, and they have less resistance to disease. The digestion and metabolism is variable and changeable, hence they cannot form sturdy and stable tissues. Their life span is usually shorter than other individuals. Because of this variable nature, they cannot perform their tasks steadily and continuously. Hence they may fail in achieving their goals or become involved in sidetracks to them.

Such individuals require a job with less strenuous physical activity, where constant attention is not required, and which is not in a cold or dry atmosphere. If they are forced to undertake such work, they are likely to become subject to diseases of the nerves and bones, and to suffer from constipation, along with loss of weight.

Pitta Constitution

These persons have quick and rapid digestive and metabolic activity. Hence they require constant food and drinks which are cool and unctuous in nature. They are able to convert food to a good quality of tissue, but as the total conversion rate in the body is very fast they also usually have shorter life spans when compared to Kapha types. They have soft, oily, and smooth skin. They tend to become bald at an early age and their hair becomes gray prematurely. They have moderate strength and capacity to work although they are hot tempered. They have good grasping power and are very intelligent. They usually possess good knowledge in their chosen subjects, are creative in nature, and often possess wealth and status in society.

These persons require a job in a cool atmosphere, with some creative activity and intelligent work.

Kapha Constitution

These persons possess hefty, robust and thick body frames, with stout musculature. They naturally possess good strength, immunity and vitality, and are thus generally healthy and have a longer life span. They have smooth and deep voices and are often good looking. The total digestive and metabolic rate in these individuals is very slow, hence they require less food or drink. They are of a calm and quiet nature.

Kapha types can carry out work that is heavy or strenuous. They are also good in maintaining public relations. However, they should not work in cold and damp atmospheres. They are likely to become obese and may fall victim to joint diseases and heart problems.

PHYSICAL CONSTITUTION

This is decided according to the dominance of the elements at the time of union of the sperm and ovum. These are variations on the humoral constitutions, as usually Kapha is watery, Pitta fiery, and Vata airy. Earthy constitution is generally categorized under Kapha and etheric under Vata.

Earthy (Parthiva) constitutions have a body which is bulky, heavy, square, and thick. The bones are usually large and there may be a significant amount of body hair. Etheric (Akashiya) constitutions have lightness and looseness, and the body has clear senses and open external orifices.

PSYCHOLOGICAL CONSTITUTION

This is decided according to which of the three gunas is dominant at the time of birth, though being a mental factor it can be more easily changed by life-activity and learning.

Sattvic Constitution

These individuals possess a good intellect and memory, and have an inherent instinct for cleanliness. Although they tend to possess a great deal of knowledge, they will always make efforts to gain more. They have a good will and allow others to prosper. They are polite, have faith in the Divine and devotion to the good.

Rajasic Constitution

Rajasic types have a nature that tries to overpower others. They manifest a propulsive and dynamic energy. They are not satisfied with the positions and possessions they achieve, and therefore always strive for more. Hence they are ambitious and industrious in nature. Usually these people are hot-tempered and egoistic. They over-express pain or pleasure. They have a brave but jealous and cruel character.

Tamasic Constitution

These persons are lazy and ignorant. Similarly, they are not curious about anything. Usually they have less intelligence, prefer not to work and are interested mainly in eating and sleeping. They avoid cleanliness and are not health conscious. They are afraid of many things, hence they do not initiate any work on their own.

SATTVIC	RAJASIC	TAMASIC
Promotes knowledge by fair means	Promotes knowledge by any means	Ignorant about knowledge
Very intelligent	Average intelligence	Unintelligent
Good memory	Variable memory	Poor memory
Accepts his status and wealth; No strong desires	Strong desire for status and wealth; Ambitious and dynamic	No desire for anything, lethargic
Gives fairly to all, unselfish	Takes advantage, selfish	Selfish, non-striving
Develops purity of body, mind, and speech	Agitated in body, mind, and speech	Unclean in body, mind, & speech
Polite, joyful	Sometimes rude and angry	Sorrowful, depressed
Calm and quiet	Brave, cruel, greedy	Fearful, vile
Believes in God or Truth	Questions God or Truth	Believes in falsehood
Inherent health and conscious capacity	Follows health advice when convinced	Ignorant about health; does not follow medical advice
Reacts to pain and pleasure properly	Over-reacts to pain and pleasure	Fails to react to pleasure and pain

IMPORTANCE OF CONSTITUTION

If we observe different individuals and their nutritional requirements, their tolerance to the atmosphere, or their behavior patterns we find that for maintaining health they have different needs. They may prefer different types of food, drink, and activity. Even if two people with identical weight and height are chosen, their requirements still may be quite varied. One may prefer large amounts of food or drink, while the other may prefer less. If we analyze the serum or blood in these individuals, we may not find any substantial difference. Yet differences clearly exist.

Therefore, it becomes clear that tolerance to food, drink or environment cannot be decided by the analytical study of the body tissues. It depends upon individual constitution. By understanding the constitution of every individual, we know which food and drink and what type of job and exercise are appropriate for maintaining their health.

As there is a predominance of Dosha in each individual, each type requires substances different or opposite to the constitution to maintain health. Vata people possess qualities of coldness, dryness, roughness, and lightness. Hence a person of Vata constitution requires food which is warm or hot, oily, or unctuous. Otherwise, there is always a tendency for Vata to increase, giving rise to Vata diseases. To compensate for the Vata in his constitution, he should eat food having sweet, sour and salty tastes.

For maintenance of health, every person should know his or her constitution. We have seen that in each constitution there is a predominance of one or more humors. If the daily activities, diet, occupation, and behavior are not adjusted to balance this, then the constitutional humor will increase, thus giving rise to its characteristic diseases. If the constitution is known then herbs, diet, and other regimens including yogic postures can be advised correctly both for disease treatment and to promote longevity.

***

CONSTITUTION CHART

PHYSICAL FEATURES	VATA	PITTA	KAPHA
BODY FRAME	Lean & thin	Moderate	Large & thick
BODY WEIGHT	Low	Moderate	Overweight
SKIN	Dry, rough, cool, black, brown	Soft, oily, warm, fair, yellowish, red	Thick, oily, cool, pale, white, glistening
HAIR	Dry, rough, brittle, blackish, brown	Soft, oily, early grey, baldness, yellow, red	Thick, oily, wavy, dark, glistening, white
TEETH	Irregular, protruded, crooked, thin gums, tendency toward tooth decay	Regular, moderate, soft gums, yellowish	Regular, strong, white, healthy

PHYSICAL FEATURES	VATA	PITTA	KAPHA
EYES	Small, dull, attractive, brown, black iris	Medium, sharp, penetrating, green, grey, yellowish iris	Big, blue iris, thick eyelashes
JOINTS	Bony markings seen	Just visible	Not seen
MUSCULATURE	Slender but hard	Loose	Firm, stout
APPETITE	Variable, scanty	Good, excessive	Low but steady
THIRST	Variable	Excessive	Less
SWEATING	Variable	Excessive	Less
SLEEP	Scanty, interrupted	Moderate, 4-6 hours slightly disturbed	More than 6 hours sound
TASTE	Sweet, sour, salty	Sweet, bitter, astringent	Pungent, bitter, astringent
ELIMINATION	Irregular, dry, hard, constipated	Regular, soft, oily, loose	Regular, oily
PHYSICAL ACTIVITY	Fast & very active	Medium	Lethargic & slow
SEXUAL VITALITY	Less	Moderate	Good
PULSE	Thready & weak	Jumping	Broad & slow

PSYCHOLOGICAL FUNCTIONS	VATA	PITTA	KAPHA
DREAMS	Fearful, flying, jumping, running	Fiery, anger, violence, war	Watery, rivers, oceans, swimming, romantic
EMOTIONAL TEMPERAMENT	Unpredictable, anxious, insecure	Irritable, aggressive, greedy, jealous	Calm, quiet
MIND	Restless, active	Aggressive, intelligent	Calm
FAITH	Changeable	Fanatic	Steady
MEMORY	Recent good, remote poor	Sharp	Slow but prolonged

PSYCHOLOGICAL FUNCTIONS

	VATA	PITTA	KAPHA
INTERESTS	Recreation, dance, drama, cultural activities	Dress and ornaments	Philosophical topics

ADVICE ON FOOD AND BEHAVIOR ACCORDING TO CONSTITUTION

	VATA	PITTA	KAPHA
FRUIT	Sweet Fruit, Bananas, Coconut, Apples, Fresh Figs, Grapefruit, Grapes, Mango, Sweet Melons, Oranges, Papaya, Peaches, Pineapples, Plums, Berries, Cherries	Sweet Fruit, Apples, Avocadoes, Coconut, Figs, Sweet Melons, Sweet Oranges, Pears, Pineapples, Plums, Pomegranate, Prunes	Apples, Apricots, Berries, Cherries, Dry Figs, Mango, Peaches, Pears, Raisins, Prunes
VEGETABLES	Cooked, Asparagus, Beets, Carrots, Garlic, Cooked Onion, Radishes, Spinach, Sprouts, Sweet Potato, Tomatoes, Zucchini	Sweet & Bitter, Asparagus, Cabbage, Cucumber, Cauliflower, Celery, Green Beans, Lettuce, Peas, Parsley, Potatoes, Sprouts, Zucchini	Pungent & Bitter, Beets, Cabbage, Carrots, Cauliflower, Celery, Eggplant, Garli c, Lettuce, Mushrooms, Onions, Parsley, Peas, Radishes, Spinach, Sprouts

ADVICE ON FOOD AND BEHAVIOR ACCORDING TO CONSTITUTION

	VATA	PITTA	KAPHA
GRAINS	Oats (cooked) Rice Wheat	Barley Oats (cooked) Rice (basmati) Rice (white) Wheat	Barley Corn Millet Oats (dry) Rice (basmati) (small amount) Rye

ANIMAL FOODS
(Note: Ayurveda recommends a vegetarian diet because of its sattvic properties, but includes animal foods for those who take them)

	VATA	PITTA	KAPHA
	Beef Chicken or Turkey(white meat) Eggs (fried or scrambled) Seafood	Chicken or Turkey(white meat) Eggs (white) Rabbit	Chicken or Turkey(dark meat) Eggs (not fried or scrambled) Rabbit
LEGUMES	No legumes except Mung Beans	All legumes except Lentils	All legumes are good except Kidney Beans, Soy Beans, Black Lentils
NUTS	All Nuts in small quantities	No Nuts	No Nuts at all
SWEETENERS	Jaggery, Raw Sugar	Raw sugar, No Honey	Only Honey and Jaggery
CONDIMENTS	All spices good, with heavy food	No spices exceptCoriander, Fennel, Cardamom, Cinnamon, Turmeric and a small amount of Black Pepper	All spices good, with light food

ANIMAL FOODS

	VATA	PITTA	KAPHA
DAIRY	Ghee Fresh Butter Milk Cottage Cheese	Butter (unsalted) Cottage cheese Ghee Milk	Milk in small quantity Goat's milk
OILS	All oils are good, particularly Sesame	Coconut Olive Sunflower Soy	No oils except Almond, Corn, or Sunflower in small amounts
LIFE-STYLE INSTRUCTIONS	Avoid fasting, Avoid strong, frequent exercise & heavy work; Avoid air-conditioned atmosphere; Avoid too much traveling	Avoid using pickles, vinegar, chilies,ketchup, canned food, aerated drinks and alcohol; Do not work at night	Avoid sleeping in day time, Avoid eating frozen or cold food; Avoid sedentary jobs near hot furnaces, or factories of synthetic chemicals and petroleum products
YOU ARE PRONE TO THE FOLLOWING DISEASES	Nerve pain, arthritis and joint problems, rectal prolapse, fissures on palms and soles, hysteria, epilepsy	Hyperacidity, peptic ulcers, bleeding tendencies, liver diseases, hypertension	Diabetes, urinary stones, asthma, colds, cough, obesity, coronary heart disease
RECOMMENDATIONS	Apply sesame oil on the body; Use medicated enema (basti)	Donate blood; Apply sandalwood oil on skin	Apply mustard oil on the skin and massage; Regular exercise
REJUVENATIVE MEDICINES, RASAYANAS	Ashwagandha Bala Garlic Licorice	Shatavari Amalaki Chyavanprash	Haritaki Triphala Pippali Shilajit

AGGRAVATION OF THE DOSHAS AND THEIR MANAGEMENT

The key to all Ayurvedic treatment is in knowing the imbalance of the humors and how to treat them. For this we must be able to determine the factors which aggravate them, recognize the symptoms of their aggravated state, and prescribe those countermeasures which alleviate them.

VATA

Causes of High Vata

Vata becomes vitiated due to cold climate, air-conditioning, drinking cold substances like ice water, refrigerated foods or foods cold in potency like green salads. It is also vitiated by food that is dry, rough or light, like barley, millet or corn. Excessive physical exercise, particularly of a strongly aerobic nature, as well as improper movements of the body aggravate Vata, as does mental and emotional stress and strain.

Symptoms of High Vata

These are indicated by a strong desire for warm food and climate, as well as for warm clothing. Physical symptoms are constipation, lack of energy, loss of sleep, fatigue, emaciation, abdominal distention with flatulence, blackish discoloration of feces and urine, defective sensory functioning. Psychological symptoms arise like fear, anxiety, insecurity, confusion, and irrelevant talking.

Management of Vata

Treatment of Vata is divided into two types based on whether the cause is malnutrition (Dhatukshaya) or obstruction in the channels (Srotorodha).

For malnutrition the best therapy is tonification (Brimhana). Anti-Vata diet should be given after making certain that the digestive fire is in good condition. Otherwise stimulant or digestion-promoting herbs should be given like dry ginger, cayenne or black pepper. Then light oil massage should be given with warm oils like sesame and fomentation with anti-Vata herbs like Dashamula or rasna. Sudation or sweating therapy with moist heat is essential. Herbal wines should be taken before food to increase appetite, or after food as a tonic. Draksha or Ashwagandha herbal wine are best. Sitting-type yoga postures with silent meditation are helpful.

For obstruction in the channels, detoxifying and stimulating herbs should be taken like dry ginger or fennel. Oil massage should use herbs like Nirgundi or Vishagarbha oil. Special alkali medicines may be taken internally to open the channels. Mild laxatives and decoction enemas should be taken. Herbal wines prepared with jaggery and herbs like rasna and Dashamula should be given. When the system is clean, then anti-Vata diet and tonifying methods can be taken.

PITTA
Causes of High Pitta

Pitta is aggravated by food that is hot in temperature, or by hot potency food like chili, black pepper, and mustard, or by too much fried food. Working on night shifts, hot environments or excessive exposure to the sun also increase Pitta. Psychological factors are anger, irritability and hot temper.

Symptoms of High Pitta

These are desire for cold food, cool environment and cool clothing. Physical symptoms are excessive hunger and thirst, burning sensation in the skin, eyes, or hands. Hypersensitivity may develop in the form of allergic rashes, fevers or giddiness. There is yellowish discoloration of the skin, eyes, urine, and feces. Psychological factors of anger, rage, hatred, and jealousy increase. Many inflammatory diseases can arise.

Management of Pitta

Anti-Pitta diet should be taken with sweet, bitter, and astringent tastes. This includes dairy products like milk, butter and ghee, mung beans, basmati rice, wheat, all sweet fruits, and cool spices like coriander. Bathing or swimming in cool water should be done, followed by light massage with coconut or sandalwood oil. Aromas like rose can be used, like rose water application in the nose. Purgation and blood-letting can be done in more serious conditions. Cool colors like blue, white and purple, and cool gems like sapphire and pearl are good.

KAPHA
Causes of High Kapha

Dietary factors are cold, oily and heavy foods like yogurt, cheese, butter, milk and meat, as well as watery fruits and vegetables like cucumber, melons, oranges, and grapes. Whole grains like wheat and rice in excess also increase Kapha. Cold and damp environments or work situations are additional factors. Psychological factors are greed and attachment.

Symptoms of High Kapha

These are loss of appetite, nausea and possible vomiting, heaviness in the body, pallor of the skin, cold hands and feet, swollen joints, cough with phlegm, excessive sleep, lethargy, and lack of concentration.

Management of Kapha

The person should carry out strong exercise. Deep massage should be done with light and dry oils like mustard. Strong dry sweating or saunas should be taken. Anti-Kapha diet should be taken with dry and hot food, with pungent, bitter, and astringent tastes. For increasing digestion ginger, black pepper, and turmeric should be used. Therapeutic vomiting can be given in severe cases.

4
THE AYURVEDIC
APPROACH TO HEALTH

Ayurveda is not just a system of medicine but a science of health promotion designed to increase our well-being and happiness in all aspects. It shows us not only how to treat disease but how to live in such a way as to arrive at optimum health and the maximum utilization of our faculties, which according to Yoga and Ayurveda are almost unlimited.

AYURVEDIC REGIMEN FOR OPTIMAL HEALTH

Maintenance of a healthy life by one's own right action is called "Swasthavritta," which literally means "the regime of abiding in one's own nature." According to the Ayurvedic science of life and the Yogic science of Self-realization, harmony is our natural state. Yet to maintain this condition we must know our nature and learn to live according to its real needs. This is the key to health. It is this science of self-care that teaches us to live healthily and happily until death.

In order to achieve a healthy and happy life, each one of us should observe certain disciplines or duties. They are:

- Daily regimen
- Seasonal regimen
- Occasional duties
- Precautionary observances in sexual activity
- General rules of conduct for the well-being of society
- Precautionary measures against untimely old-age
- Conduct and practices to achieve Self-realization

The Ayurvedic regime of right living is designed for maintenance of health, achievement of a long, healthy, active life, providing relief from pain and disease, allowing satisfactory enjoyment of the pleasures of life, and attainment of Self-realization. In short, Ayurveda helps the individual to achieve the four main objectives of human life. These are Dharma, service to society; Artha, service to family; Kama, service to self; and Moksha, Self-realization.

Optimal Health (Swastha)

A person whose bodily Doshas (Vata, Pitta, Kapha) are in a state of equilibrium, with balanced digestion and metabolism (Agni), in whom the functions of the tissues and waste materials are normal and accompanied by properly functioning senses and a happy state of being, is a truly healthy individual.

If Swastha or the healthy state is maintained from birth and the three Doshas remain in a balanced state, then the person achieves a well-formed constitution, attractive appearance, good muscular strength, and complete peace of mind.

Good health can be maintained until death. For this, one should intelligently follow all the rules laid down according to this science. Only then only will a person enjoy an optimum life span of a hundred years without contracting disease. He will also gain recognition in society, friendship with all people, and honor and wealth as he has the energy and ability to achieve all the goals of life.

The ancient Ayurvedic teacher Vagbhatta supports this view. To achieve a healthy condition of body, mind and soul, he has advised four rules of conduct —

- Only use those enjoyable objects and circumstances that your organs and mind are agreeably accustomed to.

- Do all things properly after repeatedly thinking about their adaptability to yourself.

- Maintain a habit of always criticizing your own actions intelligently.

- Always use things that balance your constitution and the season, whereby physical ease is maintained.

Ideal Healthy Person

According to Sushruta, the ideal healthy person is an individual who has a balanced constitution. People who have a balanced condition from birth are able to digest the correct amount of food and maintain proper elimination. Their systems and organs function normally and they have a happy state of mind.

SIGNS OF LONGEVITY

Vagbhatta and Charaka have explained the visible physical signs of longevity at length.

The skin of the individual is soft, smooth, firm, and fine. The forehead is prominent with the shape of a half-moon. The ears, when viewed from the front, appear small, but appear large, raised up, and full of flesh when seen from behind.

The eyes show their white and black parts distinctly. The eyelashes are thick and well set. The nose is straight and moderately prominent, with the end raised up somewhat and large nostrils. The lips are red but not protruding. The jaws are large, as is the mouth. The teeth touch each other and are glossy, smooth, white in color, and equal in size. The tongue is red, long, and thin. The chin is big and well-formed. The nails are thin, red, and raised up slightly. The hands and feet are rather large, glossy, full of flesh, and reddish. The fingers are long and when placed together do not leave any space between them.

The back of the body is expansive and the spine covered with flesh. The voice is deep and resonant, with a nasal sound to it, and lingers after speaking. The skin is glossy and vibrant. All the bones are appropriately proportioned and capable of separate and easy movement. The joints are well-knit and strongly connected by muscle and blood, strong and full of flesh. The flesh and blood are of the best quality, in the right proportion, and all the limbs are ideally juxtaposed.

Such individuals of proportionate musculature and compactness of the body possess very good strength. Hence they can defend themselves from the onslaught of disease. They can stand hunger, thirst, heat of the sun, cold, and severe physical exercise. They can digest and assimilate large amounts of food properly.[1]

Tissue Excellence (Dhatu Sara)

Individuals with good longevity possess additional signs of their tissues being in optimal states.

The optimal condition of the plasma (Rasa Dhatu) is evidenced by the qualities of skin, which is glossy, smooth, soft, attractive, thin, and tender.

When the blood (Rakta Dhatu) is in optimal condition and all the parts of the body like the ears, mouth, tongue, lips, nose, palms, and soles of the feet are glossy and red in color.

When the muscle tissue (Mamsa Dhatu) is in optimal condition the back of the neck, forehead, temples, eyes, chin, shoulders, stomach, breasts, and joints of the hands and feet become solid, strong, attractive, and full of flesh.

When the fat tissue (Meda Dhatu) is in optimal condition it causes the skin to be glossy and fine, the eyes bright and attractive, the voice deep and pleasing, and the hair and nails soft and glossy.

When the bone tissue (Asthi Dhatu) is in optimal condition, the person has large and well-formed heels, ankles, knees, elbows, collar bones, chin, and forehead. The other bones, nails, and teeth are large, compact, and steady.

When the nerve tissue (Majja Dhatu) is in optimal condition, one possesses a very soft but strong body, deep voice, glossy skin, and long and rounded joints.

When the reproductive tissue (Shukra Dhatu) is in optimal condition, one possesses an attractive personality, joyful temperament, glossy and strong teeth, hair and nails, large red lips, and a good sexual capacity.

***

Measurement of Body Proportion

The individual finger unit is called anguli pramana. The height of an average healthy individual is eighty-four times the finger breadth. This means that if the average finger breadth is 2 centimeters the height should be 168 centimeters or about 5'6". The calculation of finger breadth is done by taking the extent of both palms at the metacarpo-phalangial joints divided by eight (as this width together is the average for eight fingers).

Life Span

The optimal life span of the human being is one hundred years, which is divided into three stages:

- Youth is from birth to the age of 30 (the immature stage from birth to 16 and the mature stage from 16 to 30).

- Middle age is from 31 to 60 years.

- Old is age from 61 to 100 years.

Longevity depends upon many factors but the most important is Prakriti or constitution. Individuals of either Kapha or balanced constitution live longer. If in addition they have good Ojas and excellence of all tissues (Dhatu Sara), they can live up to an age of 120. For such longevity it is presumed that the individual follows the disciplines described in Swasthavritta.

Physical Indications of Long Life

In *Charaka Samhita* the signs of longevity, as evidenced in children, are described:

ORGANS	FEATURES INDICATING LONGEVITY
Hair	Discrete, soft, sparse, oily, firmly rooted, and lustrous
Skin	Thick and firm
Head	Larger than normal in size, firmly rooted, and lustrous
Forehead	Broad, strong, even, having firm union with temporal bones, and with three transverse lines, in appearance like a half moon
Ears	Thick, large in size with even lobes, equal in size and elongation downwards with big ear cavities
Eyes	Equal in size, having clear cut division between pupil and sclera, strong, lustrous and beautiful
Nose	Straight, slightly curved at the tip
Tongue	Smooth, thin, red
Voice	Sweet, deep toned
Neck	Round in shape
Chest	Broad and full
Hands & Arms	Round, full, and extended
Thighs	Tapering downward, round and plump[2]

In addition Charaka explains forty-seven factors for ascertaining the span of life including examination of sense organs, mind (desire, purity, conduct, behavior, memory, intelligence), and characteristic features of disease.[3]

IMMUNITY

Immunity is the power of the body to prevent the development of disease or to resist a disease that has developed. This definition is generally applicable to infectious as well as non-infectious diseases. Yet all bodies do not have the same power of resistance against all diseases. Persons who are too heavy, flaccid, or fat or those who are too lean or thin, whose blood, bones and muscles are not well developed, who take an unbalanced or deficient diet, or who are weak or nervous, have a lower power to resist disease. Individuals with opposite qualities to these are better able to resist disease. Ayurveda believes that if the body is kept perfectly healthy and its strength is maintained at its best, there can be little chance of its falling prey even to very contagious diseases.

In Ayurveda, the strength of the body (bala) has two main aspects — physical strength (Vyayamashakti) and the power of resistance to disease (Vyadhikshamatwa). The factors which maintain and promote the strength or the natural resistance of the body are contributed by good quality tissues like plasma, blood, reproductive tissue, Kapha and Ojas. Resistance to disease is classified under three main types.

Natural (Sahaja)	that which is inborn or genetic and exists from birth
Temporal (Kalaja)	that which is under the influence of time, such as seasonal changes and the person's age
Developed (Yuktikrit)	that produced by right action in life by resorting to appropriate food, sleep and rest, control of sexual energy, and use of rejuvenative therapy (Rasayana)

For the prevention of disease, Ayurveda stresses the maintenance and promotion of the natural defence mechanism of the body by the observance of Swasthavritta, the rules of health and self-care.

The biological humors are always in a state of flux or shifting equilibrium. Hence they should be adjusted to ever changing environmental factors as these factors may initiate the disease process. Therefore, for maintenance of optimal health, even transient disturbances should not be allowed to go unnoticed.

If a person follows the prescribed regimen of life as described in Swasthavritta, he or she can attain full longevity and remain healthy throughout life. Ayurveda advises three important regimens for this purpose:

- Daily regimen (Dinacharya)
- Seasonal regimen (Ritucharya)
- Ethical regimen (Sadvritta)

Similarly, Ayurveda gives much attention to diet, sleep and sexual intercourse.

∗ ∗ ∗

AYURVEDIC HEALTH REGIMENS
I. DAILY REGIMEN

Ayurveda outlines the main practices to be done on a daily basis to promote optimal health and optimal usage of our faculties. These practices should be done by everyone.

Time to Wake Up

A healthy person should arise two hours before sunrise. After attending to the calls of nature and evacuation of the bowels, one should meditate for half an hour and then carry out Yoga exercises including Pranayama, emphasizing postures (Asanas) which are appropriate for one's constitution as follows:

Vata	Lotus pose, Vajrasana, Siddhasana, Alternate nostril breathing in through the right and out through the left nostril (Solar Pranayama)
Pitta	Plow pose (Halasana), Shoulder stand, Shitali Pranayama
Kapha	Pashchimotasana, Neti, and Agnisara

Care of the Teeth

The teeth should be cleaned with medicated powders mixed with oil and salt. The mouth is the place of Bodhaka Kapha and has an alkaline PH. Hence the teeth should be brushed or, better yet, cleaned with the fingers, with medicated powders containing astringent, bitter and slightly pungent taste substances. For this purpose, a mixture of the powder of catechu, rock salt, black pepper, long pepper, camphor, turmeric, and neem in equal proportions, along with a small amount of cloves and honey is recommended.

Such Ayurvedic tooth powders are commercially available. They often use a base of natural astringent and antiseptic clays, along with various spicy and astringent herbs. If used regularly, they can eliminate many dental problems, particularly gum diseases which are the main cause of tooth loss. Their taste, however, is often strong and make take some getting used to. Ayurvedic toothpastes are also available which are quite pleasant. They use such herbs in extract form as part of the toothpaste.

Care of the Tongue

The tongue should be cleaned by a flexible and long strip of metal or wood. Steel or copper are used for this purpose. Copper also has antiseptic properties but it does tarnish. Each person should use a tongue scraper every day. Clearing the tongue not only cleanses the mouth but also stimulates the whole digestive tract and improves the digestive fire. Failing to clean the tongue in the morning is considered in Ayurveda as equal to not washing the face.

Care of the Mouth

Gargling with 1/4 cup warm undiluted sesame oil is recommended. This gives strength to the teeth, improves the voice, and imparts proper taste to the food that is eaten.

Care of the Face

Every morning the face and eyes should be washed with cool water. A medicated paste containing haritaki, sandalwood, and milk should be applied to the face and kept on for ten minutes. Then it should be washed with water. This paste is a little astringent and helps tighten the skin and prevent wrinkling. Other herbal and facial oils can similarly be used, like Brahmi oil.

An Ayurvedic facial paste can be made with 1 part amalaki powder, 1/2 part haritaki powder, and 1/4 part sandalwood powder. This should be mixed with two or three tablespoons of milk until it becomes a paste.

Care of the Eyes

Every day collyrium or kajjal should be put into the eyes. This helps remove dirt and dust, and relieves watering or burning of the eyes due to strain. Regular use of collyrium increases the brightness of the eyes and strengthens their ability to withstand bright light. Collyrium should be made from the decoction of barberry, licorice, and Triphala in equal parts along with enough honey to produce a paste. This can be applied into the eyes.

For making collyrium the best substance is the ash from a ghee lamp. To make this a copper or silver bowl with a small amount of water in it is held over a ghee lamp. The black soot which accumulates under the bowl is collected as collyrium.

Medicated ghee made with the Triphala formula is also good for oil application to the eyes.

Care of the Nose

Medicated oil should be put into both nostrils every day (this is called Pratimarsha Nasya). A few drops can be put on the end of the little finger and gently applied into the nose. For this purpose the Ayurvedic oil called Anu Tail should be used or, if it is not available, such oils as sesame oil, Brahmi oil, or ghee are also helpful. Constant use of Nasya protects the eyes, nose, and throat against disease and improves their efficiency. It is also helps prevent diseases of the neck and head region and strengthens the voice.

Massage

Rubbing of the body is called massage. This can be done by the fingers, palms of the hand, or even the feet. Different degrees of pressure can be applied by kneading or by vibration techniques. Proper massage removes fatigue, increases muscular tone and flexibility of joints, alleviates Vata, improves blood circulation of different organs and skin, eliminates waste products through the skin, stimulates the nervous system, prevents old age and increases longevity.

Different alternative health-care systems use different substances for massage, including various medicated oils, herbal pastes or powders, pieces of brick, wood, metal balls, or sand. In adition to oil massage, Ayurveda specifies four types of massage each utilizing different substances to enhance its beneficial effects.

Oil Massage

Oil massage is known in Sanskrit as Abhyanga. Medicated oil should be massaged on the whole body, including the head and feet. Regular oil massage removes excess fat from the skin, makes the skin glossy, soft, and strengthens it. It also protects the skin from diseases. Persons of Vata constitution should use medicated oils prepared from demulcent herbs like shatavari, ashwagandha, or bala (like Narayana oil) and it should be applied while the oil is warm. Persons of Pitta constitution should apply medicated oils using sandalwood or vetivert (like Chandabalalakshadi). Those of Kapha constitution should use oils prepared from substances like mustard, saffron, and agaru. As a result of oil massage health is preserved, disease is prevented, and immunity increased.

By massaging oil to the head regularly, premature hair loss or greying of the hair is prevented, and sound sleep is also promoted. By massaging oil to the soles of the feet and to the legs, the eyesight is improved, cracks to the skin of the feet are prevented, and the reproductive system is also strengthened.

Other Types of Ayurvedic Massage

UDVARTANA MASSAGE is done with different ointments and powders that remove the oils which have been applied on the body during oil massage. Powders of horsegram, chick pea, or mung flour are used for this. It is also a routine procedure done after Abhyanga or oil massage.

UDGHARSHANA MASSAGE is done with dry powder of herbs that will provoke heat and open the pores of the sweat glands on the skin. This can also be done by using sand. Powders of calamus, lodhra, and shikai are used. Calamus is best for small children. This massage also helps to remove excess fat under the skin and cures vitiation of Kapha. It is one of the main treatment measures for obesity.

UTSADANA MASSAGE is done with pieces of brick, small cuttle-fish bone, or wood sticks. It is also used for removing excess oil from the skin after Abhyanga or oil massage.

ANNALEPANA MASSAGE is done with medicated boiled rice. First the rice is cooked along with the husk. Then milk is boiled with Dashamula and small balls of cooked rice are put into it. These are taken out and used for massage in a cloth bag with about two hands full of rice in each cloth bag. First oil massage is done and then massage is done with rice in a direction from above downward, below the head. Then massage is done on the chest, back, hands, and legs. Then the rice paste is removed and hot oil is applied again. After removing the excess oil, a hot water bath should be taken.

Exercise

Regular light exercise should be done by everybody. With exercise the body grows and becomes proportionate in shape. Muscular strength increases. The body comes to withstand exertion, fatigue, heat, and cold. The appetite also is improved and health is maintained. Exercise is most beneficial in the winter and spring seasons. It is best when done to the extent of half the exercising capacity. When sweat appears on the forehead and armpits, and respiration becomes quick and one is forced to breathe by opening the mouth, these are the signs that exercise should be stopped.

While doing any exercise, due consideration must be given to age, strength, physical condition, time, season of the year, and diet. If exercise is done without paying attention to these factors, or if too much exercise is done, then it aggravates Vata and the blood, and produces many diseases. Similarly individuals suffering from diseases or who are too old, debilitated and exhausted should not undertake any strong exercise.

Western and Yogic Exercise

Yogic and Western types of exercises, when studied in comparison to each other, appear to have different effects. Strong contraction and relaxation for the achievement of good muscular build and power is the aim of most Western styles of physical culture. Yogic exercise, on the other hand, gives more importance to a posture achieved and maintained with the least stressful movement. Similarly, exertions that require quick and short breathing are not recommended, while slower and longer breathing is advised, as such breathing aids in longevity.

According to Ayurveda, exercise should be stopped when one has to breathe in and out quickly, when there is a sensation of dryness in the mouth, and when perspiration appears on the forehead. Exercise done with such restriction is said to be of optimum use. If exercise is stopped at this stage one can prevent bodily secretions and exudations from leaving the gastro-intestinal tract and adversely affecting other bodily sites. The Western style of exercise, on the other hand, emphasizes the need of "warming up," which is indicated when perspiration appears on the forehead, and does not stop the exercise at this point.

Skeletal muscular exertions can cause hepatic, splenic, or mesenteric reserves to empty themselves into the peripheral circulation. This may lead to a movement of undigested products into the tissues resulting in disease. Therefore the ideal exercise according to Ayurveda is based on the understanding of central and peripheral activity of the Doshas or biological humors. Ayurvedic exercise lays emphasis on lightness of the body. Versatility to flex, bend or extend is another quality that is desired. Firmness but not rigidity or hardness in the architecture of the skeletal tissue is the goal. Evaluation of physical ability is not based on the size of the individual muscle or the "body beautiful" but the capacity to withstand heat, cold, hunger, thirst, or fatigue. Indian thought considers Yoga the best means of achieving the greatest physical ability. The initial stages of Yogic exercise and discipline lay emphasis also on the restriction of diet and behavior which leads to purification of the body.

Smoking

Smoking a cigarette made of medicinal herbs (without tobacco) is useful for alleviating Kapha in the neck and head region. This type of smoking is also helpful for maintaining health and treating certain diseases.

Medicinal herbs and substances used for smoking are harenu, priyangu, keshar, sandalwood, cinnamon leaf, cardamom, licorice, jatamansi, guggul, agaru, udumbara, ashwattha, plaksha, lodhra, cyperus, resin of Vateria indica, lotus, resinous extract from Pinus roxburghii, and shallaki. All these herbs should be powdered and then made into a paste and applied to a reed. Then they are made into a cigarette having the thickness of the center of the thumb and the length of eight fingers breadth. It should then be dried up and the reed taken out. Then with the help of a cigarette holder one can smoke the cigarette after greasing it with an oily substance like sesame oil.

Smoking can be done after taking a bath, after lunch or dinner, after brushing the teeth, after applying collyrium to the eyes, or just after getting up from bed in the morning. Smoking should not be done after drinking alcohol, when the body is rough and dry, when there is a severe headache, or injury to the head.

Smoking should be done through the mouth but smoke should not be exhaled through the nose because this can irritate the eyes. Effects of correct and good smoking are lightness in the head, throat and chest since it liquefies excess Kapha in these regions.

Bath

A hot water bath should be taken after oil massage and proper exercise. For washing the head the water should not be too hot.

Hot water bath relieves fatigue, increases strength, cleans the body, improves appetite and imparts a pleasant sensation to the body as well as the mind.

Rest and Sleep

Before going to bed meditation should be practiced and one should critically examine his own conduct. Usually six to seven hours sleep gives sufficient rest to both body and mind.

***

II. SEASONAL REGIMEN

It is a well known fact that different atmospheric changes take place due to changes of season. These changes in the atmosphere affect all living beings. Some changes are beneficial, while others are detrimental. In order to achieve maximum benefits from the good qualities of the atmosphere and protection from the bad effects, Ayurveda has prescribed certain rules — in regard to diet, behavior, and medicines — called "seasonal regimen" or Ritucharya.

All the activities in the universe are governed by two energy principles, hot and cold. Based on this concept the entire time span of the year has been divided into two parts, accumulation (Adana) and release (Visarga). In India they follow the northern course of the sun (Uttarayana), the period from the winter to the summer solstice, and the southern course of the Sun (Dakshinayana), the period from the summer to the winter solstice. In the Adana (taking) period, nature takes away energy and strength from all living beings, whereas during the Visarga (giving) period, nature gives energy and strength to all living beings.

During the accumulation period (Adana) the increasing heat of the Sun imparts hot and dry qualities to living beings as well as to plants.

During this period, the green grass supply is scanty and consequently animal products and dairy products are not supplied sufficiently. Their quality is not very nutritious either. Due to extreme heat, the natural decomposition of food stuff is faster. This increasing heat reduces the strength of all individuals and also lowers the appetite. The grains, vegetables, or herbs that grow during this period have predominantly bitter, pungent, and astringent tastes. The incidence of disease is more frequent.

During the release (Visarga) period, there is a dominance of the moon and the principle of cold. Hence the strength of creatures increases along with their appetite. In plants, predominatly sour, salty, and sweet tastes are found. As immunity or resistance to diseases increases during this period, people at large do not suffer from diseases and their health is maintained. The food that is available during this period is also more nourishing since the natural process of decay is not as fast as it is in the extreme hot season. As a result of this, the whole environment enhances the possibilities of better tissue building.

While discussing seasonal schedules, one should understand the priniple on which the entire pattern is based. Change in the environmental factor (hot or cold) is a stimulus for all living beings. To compensate for this stimulus, a modification in the response pattern is essential. This is called the seasonal regimen. The division of seasons depends on the actual meteorological conditions in each place. In India we have six divisions, but in other countries there may be as few as two different seasons in the whole year.

The substances that are advised for a particular period must also be understood according to their qualities (the three gunas, five elements, and twenty attributes). In general the substances to be selected in a particular season should have qualities opposite the season. If this rule is not followed, then these substances can have adverse effects.

We have seen that seasonal variations affect the human body and mind. Due to changes in season, changes in the Doshas also take place, like accumulation, aggravation, and subsidence. If the diet, mode of living, and routine are not adjusted so as to keep the equilibrium of the Doshas, diseases are certain to occur.

The Doshic fluctuations caused by seasonal variations have considerable significance in the prevention of seasonal diseases. In India we have six seasons, each of two months duration. Vata is provoked during the rainy season, Pitta in autumn, and Kapha in spring. Therefore, one should not indulge in things like foods and acts which are likely to increase or provoke the respective Doshas. On the other hand, one should resort to

Vamana or herb induced emesis in early winter, Virechana or herb induced purgation in autumn and Basti or medicated enema in the rainy season to eliminate Kapha, Pitta, and Vata respectively. By carrying out these measures, one can prevent seasonal diseases.

For temperate climates the Kapha season is early spring, Pitta is summer, and Vata late autumn. During the seasons their respective purification therapies should be employed.

✳ ✳ ✳

III. ETHICAL REGIMEN

A healthy mind is as important as a healthy body. The mind influences many physiological actions. When the body possesses a Sattvic quality of mind, it directs all desires and actions for the welfare of an individual. Rajas and Tamas are harmful qualities of mind, and are produced by passions and ignorant actions. Such an unhealthy mind generates wrong judgments and misconceptions by the intellect and is responsible for producing diseases. Hence every attempt should be made to increase the Sattvic quality of the mind.

Ayurveda prescribes certain rules for maintaining a healthy state of mind. They are called the "Ethical Regimen" (Sadvritta). These are not simply moral principles that reflect a particular cultural bias. They are the principles of right conduct that are applicable to all people of all times and places. Practicing them gives balance and peace to the mind. Violating or ignoring them makes us agitated in our thoughts and feelings. These are:

- Always speak the truth
- Do not lose your temper under any circumstances
- Do not get addicted to sensory pleasures
- Do not harm anyone
- As far as possible do not expose yourself to hardships
- Try to control your passions
- Endeavor to speak pleasant and sweet words
- Meditate every day for tranquility of mind
- Observe cleanliness in all things
- Be patient
- Observe self-control
- Try to distribute knowledge, good advice, and money to others
- Whenever possible devote your services to God, to wise and respectable individuals, or the elderly

- Be straightforward and kind
- Avoid irregularity in daily activities
- Consume food of Sattvic quality (Do not take overly spicy, sour, or non-vegetarian foods, or alcohol)
- Behave according to the time and place where you are residing
- Act always in a courteous and polite manner
- Control your sense organs
- Make a habit of doing all that is good and avoiding all that is bad

General Rules of Conduct

The following principles of conduct are also generally useful for everyone.

- Avoid overeating, overdrinking (alcohol), too much sexual activity, and too much or too little sleep
- Never eat food at an unhygienic place, at an improper time, or with unhealthy people
- Do not disclose another's fault or secret
- Do not take another's wealth or property
- Do not keep company with people who break the rules of good conduct
- Do not undertake strenuous work which is more than your physical capacity or when you are ill
- Do not undertake any job that is beyond your capacity
- Control all your sense organs

5
THE THREE PILLARS
OF LIFE

The key to health and disease does not lie in the application of drugs or chemicals or special therapies but in the prime factors on which our life and vitality is based. The three most important ones in Ayurveda are food, rest and sexual energy.

I. FOOD

Food sustains the life of all living beings. Complexion, clarity, good voice, longevity, genius, happiness, satisfaction, nourishment, strength, and intellect are all conditioned by food in this world, as are all practices leading to liberation from this world.

Ayurveda divides the qualities of different food articles into twelve groups: 1) grains, 2) beans, 3) meat, 4) vegetables, 5) fruit, 6) salad greens, 7) wine, 8) water, 9) dairy products, 10) cooked food preparations, 11) accessory food articles like oils and spices, 12) sugars.

We should note that although Ayurveda acknowledges the food value of meat, particularly in conditions of severe debility, it also recognizes the harm and suffering caused by eating meat. It tells us that we cannot escape the karmic consequences of eating meat unless it is something we have taken to save or protect our lives. It also acknowledges the power of meat to breed toxins and promote diseases of both body and mind. Ayurveda generally recommends a vegetarian diet but lists the properties of meat for the benefit of those who take it.

Wholesome or beneficial food quickly becomes homologous to the tissues of the body and it does not aggravate the Doshas. All herbs and foods which dislodge the Doshas but do not expel them from the body and cause vitiation of the tissues are unwholesome. Hence one should always eat wholesome food; food whose color, smell, taste and touch are pleasing to the senses and conductive to health if taken according to the rules advocated by Ayurveda. Wholesome or unwholesome food are responsible respectively for happiness (health) or misery (disease). As the body consists of food, one should take wholesome food only after careful examination and should not indulge in unwholesome food out of greed or ignorance.

The best food articles by type are as follows:

Grains	Shali (a red variety of rice which is ready in sixty days)
Legumes	Mung beans
Water	Rain water collected from high above ground level or spring water at a high altitude
Salts	Rock salt
Vegetables	Jivanti
Meat Products	Aina (a type of deer), lava (a small bird like a pigeon), and rohita (a small fish)
Dairy Products	Ghee and milk from the cow
Oils Extracted from Seeds	Sesame
Animal Fats	Pig and chicken
Fruit	Grapes

There are three special substances for alleviating the Doshas. These are sesame oil for Vata and Kapha, honey for Kapha and Vata, and ghee (clarified butter) for Pitta and Vata. Amalaki is the best herb to preserve youth. Haritaki is the best herb for removing Doshas from the body. Food sustains life, while milk strengthens life. Wine and bathing remove exhaustion.

PROPERTIES OF FOOD

All food articles are composed of three factors:

- The five elements of earth, water, fire, air, and ether
- The six tastes — sweet, sour, salty, bitter, pungent, astringent
- The twenty attributes — heavy, slow, cold, wet, sticky, dense, soft, firm, subtle, and clear, and their opposites

The combination of two elements is responsible for producing each taste as follows:

Sweet	=	Earth	+ Water	Fire	+ Air	=	Pungent
Sour	=	Fire	+ Earth	Ether	+ Air	=	Bitter
Salty	=	Fire	+ Water	Earth	+ Air	=	Astringent

Relation of the Rasas to the Doshas

The six Rasas or tastes represent six different combinations of the five elements. According to their elements they either increase or decrease the Doshas in the body. Sweet taste is produced by earth and water. Hence it will increase similar components, namely Kapha.

DECREASING	TASTE		INCREASING
VATA	Sweet, Sour, Salty		KAPHA
PITTA	Astringent : Bitter, Sweet	Pungent: Sour, Salty	PITTA
KAPHA	Bitter, Pungent, Astringent		VATA

All diets of sweet taste generally aggravate Kapha, except honey, shali rice, and barley. Usually diets of sour taste aggravate Pitta, except amalaki and pomegranate. All diets of bitter taste generally aggravate Vata and weaken sexual vitality, except guduchi, the sprouts of vetra, and the leaves of patola. Similarly all pungent articles except garlic and long pepper aggravate Vata and also weaken sexual vitality.

Qualities of Food

HEAVY (Guru) — means heavy for digestion and is connected to Brimhana or adding to the bulk of tissues. Hence all substances having sweet, astringent, and salty tastes, as well as herbs that are nutritive and restorative, aphrodisiac, and rejuvenative are heavy. This quality is found in the earth and water elements.

LIGHT (Laghu) — means light or easy for digestion. It is linked with bringing lightness or leanness to the body. Because although these are assimilated quickly, minimum tissue material is available after absorption. Substances with bitter, pungent, and sour tastes, like spices, are light in quality.

DULL (Manda) — This quality exists in earth, water, and ether. Such substances have a moderating energy or maintaining effect along with cooling and pacifying qualities as in food substances like ghee, butter, and milk.

SHARP (Tikshna) — This quality of purification is found predominantly in fire, earth, and air. Pungent taste and hot energy substances like cayenne or dry ginger are sharp.

COLD (Hima) — Coldness has an astringent property (stambhana) or obstruction to motion. Bitter, astringent, and sweet substances are cold in quality, like sandalwood. This quality (within comfortable limits) encourages health by helping all tissues to last longer and is mainly found in water.

HOT (Ushna) — On the other hand, excessive heat is not helpful to the tissues. Hot substances have the power to cause perspiration, like ginger and cinnamon. They abound in fire.

UNCTUOUS (Snigdha) — Oily substances like ghee or sesame oil have the property of rendering things wet (kledana). They also have a lubricating (Snehana) property. Oleating agents help protect the integrity of every cell.

UNUNCTUOUS (Ruksha) — This dry and dessicating quality squeezes out useful material from the cell. Such substances are barley and horse gram (kulattha), or any dry food article like toast. Hence it is not useful for tissue building.

SOFT (Slakshna) — means capable of holding fast. These substances have the quality of ropana or helping to heal. Such soft or slimy substances avoid friction and have a soothing effect as in the cases of honey or aloe gel.

ROUGH (Khara) — substances which are rough to the touch have the property to remove vitiated substances. Air predominant substances like guggul, myrrh, and alkalis are of this quality.

CONGEALING (Sandra) — Sandra is a fluid with particles in suspension. The tissue can get nourishment when a soluble solid is available. Such substances have the quality of binding things together like honey and sweet fruit juices.

LIQUEFYING (Drava) — means fluids with refreshing properties that bring about hydration of the tissues. Many liquids have this property. Pure water is not useful for building tissues unless there are certain solid substances in solution or suspension. Pure water is an example of the Drava quality, but if a pinch of salt or sugar is added to it, then it becomes Sandra.

SOFT (Mridu) — means of a pulpy quality. Fatty, oily substances are Mridu, as they have a loosening effect. They remove hardness in the body and render it soft. They contain water and earth. Examples are sesame oil, ghee or any fat.

HARD (Kathina) — Ingredients in the soft and pulpy stage (Mridu) are better assimilable as compared to those in a hard condition. All hard substances possess the property of making firm or stable. Almonds and calcium substances like coral are hard (earthy).

FIRM (Sthira) — or enduring and steady. All substances that are strengthening to the different muscles and bones have this quality, like wheat and natural calcium as found in egg shells.

MOBILE (Chala) — means unsteady or vibrating substances. They are useful in giving motion in a certain direction. If the sufficient time for assimilation is not available — if the movements are increased — it may result in tissue loss. All oily substances are mobile like almond oil, corn oil, and psyllium.

GROSS (Sthula) — Soft and round substances like butter have a covering or enveloping effect. The natural arrangement of whole substances (Sthula) is more useful than the separated or fine form (Sukshma). This is because there is a natural arrangement of bulk in gross form which aid in nutrition as well as in the excretion of waste products.

SUBTLE (Sukshma) — Alcohol, honey, and oils can spread quickly in the body because of this quality. Essential oils like wintergreen or camphor and spicy herbs abound in this quality.

STICKY (Picchila) — Sticky substances like the gums of different plants have this property of adhering or forming a coating which is useful for tissue building. Such are gum acacia, myrrh, guggul, honey, or a demulcent oil like peanut.

CLEAR (Vishada) — These are substances having the power to clean. Examples are soapnut tree, shikai, and such saponin-containing herbs as yucca root.

RULES FOR TAKING FOOD

All healthy individuals, even while eating wholesome food, should observe the rules of diet. Food must be consumed in proper quantity while it is warm and oily and it should not be contradictory in potency. It must be eaten only when the previous meal has been properly digested. Food must be taken at a clean place in the proper company of people, without too much talking or laughing and with concentration.

Warm and unctuous food is delicious in taste and it stimulates Pitta (enzymes) essential for digestion. It gets digested properly and aids the downward movement of Vata (good peristalsis). Food which is slightly oily strengthens all the sense organs and increases body strength and brightness of complexion. If it is taken in proper quantity it promotes longevity and does not impair the power of digestion.

While eating, due regard to one's own constitution should be given, and the mind should be calm and quiet. If the mind is disturbed or if there is a lot of stress and strain on the mind then appetite also gets deranged.

Indications of Proper Quantity of Food Eaten

There should be no undue pressure on the stomach or in the sides of the chest. There should not be heaviness in the abdomen, nor obstruction to the proper function of the heart. Relief from hunger and thirst, proper nourishment of the senses, as well as a comfortable feeling while walking, talking, and sleeping and increase in strength are additional signs that food has been consumed in proper quantity. All opposite signs denote that too much food has been consumed. Such food aggravates the Doshas. If it is not properly digested then Ama or toxins are produced in the gastro-intestinal tract.

Ultimately, intake of food and drink which is heavy, cold, dry, irritating or mutually contradictory, or intake of food when the individual is afflicted with passion, anger or grief produces Ama, which in turn produces disease.

Eight Factors Determining the Utility of Food

There are eight factors which determine the utility of food and are jointly responsible for its beneficial effect.

NATURE OF FOOD (Prakriti) — Each substance has its characteristic nature; for example, mutton is heavy, while rice is light. Sesame oil is damp and oily while toast is dry. In short all the qualities of food substances should be studied and applied harmoniously.

PREPARATION OF FOOD (Karana) — means the transformation of food qualities through various processes like cooking, frying, and roasting. Due to this change light substances can become heavy or vice versa.

FOOD COMBINATION (Samyoga) — Combination of foods may enhance the qualities of the original substances, or it may produce qualities other than those which are present in them. For example, the combination of fish and milk or mixing milk with sour fruit produces vitiation of blood and Pitta.

QUANTITY OF FOOD (Rashi) — This is of two types: total quantity of food consumed, and quantity of each particular article. Too much food or too much of any one food article can cause difficulties.

HABITAT WHERE FOOD IS GROWN (Desha) — The place where the food is grown and its variation of qualities according to the region, climate, and soil are important. The negative effect of modern inorganic and chemical agricultural practices should be considered here.

TIME OF EATING (Kala) — This means the time when food is consumed and the state of the individual (health or diseased) at that time. While consuming food the time of day and season should be considered. For example, heavy foods taken at night have adverse effects, as do hot foods taken in the summer.

DIETARY RULES (Upayoga Samstha) — These rules have already been described.

CONDITION OF THE PERSON EATING FOOD (Upayokta) — This means taking food according to one's constitution, that is of the appropriate nature for it and that to which one is accustomed by habitual or repeated use. The state of mind and emotions are also considered here.

WRONG OR CONTRADICTORY FOOD USAGES

Various types of food usages are not conducive to nourishment. They are said to be contradictory. Such food aggravates the Doshas but does not expel them from the body. It causes harmful effects as it is opposite to the qualities of body tissues. Charaka explains seventeen types of wrong food usages. Food taken in such ways is unwholesome and hence should not be consumed.

PLACE — Food which is wholesome in a cold region may not prove the same in a hot region. This is because of different geographical habitat. In deserts dry and pungent food should be avoided (as the climate is hot and dry), and cold and unctuous food should be avoided in marshy areas.

TIME — Cold and dry food in winter and pungent and hot food in the summer should be avoided, because weather changes require the food of opposite qualities to that of the season.

POWER OF DIGESTION — Every individual possesses a specific capacity to digest and convert food into body tissues. This capacity varies from individual to individual. Certain individuals do well avoiding heavy food, while others can be healthy only by consuming it. Here the difference is due to the individual capacity (Agni) to convert quantity and quality of food from raw to fine materials. Both types will be unhappy and unhealthy if a wrong interchange is adopted. If we consume heavy, oily, sweet food when our digestive power is low, for example, we will develop indigestion and toxins (Ama) will form.

PROPORTION OF CERTAIN FOODS — For example, honey and ghee in equal proportions is not an advisable combination.

FOOD HABIT — While advising the diet for any individual the habitual tolerance to particular foods must be taken into account. Eating sweet and cold foods for a person accustomed to pungent and hot food is not correct.

ACCORDING TO DOSHA — Usage of herbs, diet, and regimens with similar qualities to one's predominant Dosha should be avoided, such as eating dry, cold substances or fasting when Vata is aggravated.

MODE OF PREPARATION — Although individual items of food may be good, improper cooking often produces negative results.

POTENCY — Mixing substances of contradictory (cold and hot) potency together produces adverse synergism or antagonism, like milk and salt.

CONDITION OF THE GASTROINTESTINAL TRACT — This refers to the condition of the bowels. It means taking food that is too drying when there is constipation or too lubricating (laxative) when there is loose stool.

STATE OF HEALTH — For example, intake of Vata aggravating food is not advisable after exhaustion or strong physical exercise.

ORDER — Taking food before relieving an urge to evacuate the bowels.

SEQUENCE — Eating food in the wrong order, as in intake of hot and pungent things after eating pork or cold things or after eating ghee.

COOKING — The source of heat used for cooking food, i.e. gas, electricity, charcoal, etc. is very important. It may add to or subtract from the total beneficial effect of food. Similarly, methods like slow and fast heating, direct or indirect heating or baking and roasting have different beneficial effects. Undercooking or overcooking foods causes problems. A good modern example is microwaving food, which destroys its vitality (Prana).

WRONG COMBINATION — As eating sour food with milk.

PALATABILITY — Eating food which is not palatable or does not smell good or causes disgust for any reason, for it will not produce nourishment.

WRONG QUALITY — Consuming substances which are not mature will not produce beneficial results. The same occurs if we eat over-matured, preserved or even hybrid food substances. They may look wholesome but lack nutritional qualities.

RULES OF EATING — Not observing the proper rules of eating or taking meals in the wrong company.

✳ ✳ ✳

II. SLEEP

When the body gets tired and the mind turns away from the sense organs owing to the increase of the quality of Tamas in the mind, the person falls asleep. The effects of sleep are like those of diet, to provide nourishment. Just as we require proper food, so rest to the body and mind by sleep is also essential. Happiness and misery, obesity and leanness, strength and weakness, sexual vigor and impotence, consciousness and loss of sensory acuity, life and death all depend upon proper and improper sleep.

TYPES OF SLEEP

Sleep can be due to a number of causes. These are:

- Natural, due to exhaustion of mind and body
- Due to increase in Tamas or dullness in the mind
- Owing to aggravation of Kapha, which causes heaviness and fatigue
- Caused by external injury (as to the head)
- Due to diseases and the fatigue they cause
- Due to the advent of the night or according to the movement of time

Remaining awake at night provokes Pitta and causes dryness in the body; while daytime sleep provokes Kapha and increases the damp or unctuous quality in the body.

DAYTIME SLEEP

Sleep during the day is recommended for those who are old; young children; persons who are exhausted (due to wounds, operation or diseases); those suffering from indigestion, diarrhea, neuralgia, asthma, or hiccups; those tired due to travel, walking, or driving; and those who have become weak due to anger and fear. Through daytime sleep these individuals acquire balance in their physical strength and their life span is increased.

If daytime sleep is taken when not appropriate, the following symptoms or diseases occur: headache, feeling of heaviness and pain in the body, difficulty of movement, loss of movement, feeling of tightness and weakening of the heart, itching, edema, diseases of the neck, fever, and if the person has taken some poison its effects are aggravated. Daytime sleep is contraindicated for obese persons, Kapha constitutions, persons suffering from Kapha diseases or persons who have ingested poisons.

LOSS OF SLEEP (INSOMNIA)

Loss of sleep is caused by anxiety, worry, grief, anger, fear, accumulation of stress and strain, aggravation of Vata, excessive exercise, increase of Sattvic quality and decrease of Tamasic quality in the mind, and constant pressure of work.

To promote sleep, oil massage should be applied and then a hot or cold water bath. Useful practices to promote sleep are drinking wine and then eating heavy foods, meat preparations, sweets, boiled rice with milk or ghee. Singing, listening to music, joyful circumstances, the use of perfumes and flowers, and applying cooling medicines like sandalwood paste over the eyes are also good.

* * *

III. CONTROL OF SEXUAL ENERGY (BRAHMACHARYA)

Ayurveda considers Brahmacharya as the third important Pillar of Life. Brahma means knowledge or study leading to the knowledge of God, and Charya means regimen or duty. While studying, living a self-controlled life is essential. If the sense organs are properly controlled, true knowledge can be achieved during this period . This also means living a single life and observing celibacy. Vatsyana, the great Indian sexologist, has mentioned in his treatise *Kamasutra* that during Balyavastha, the period from childhood until the completion of education around twenty-one years of age, celibacy should be observed.

Brahmacharya is divided into three types: physical, which includes a regulated family life; mental or to maintain balance of mind; and spiritual, observing complete celibacy and practicing Yoga, rituals, and meditation for acquiring knowledge of God.

During adulthood, every healthy person possesses the desire for sexual intercourse. But spiritual teachings like the *Upanishads* do not look at this act from the angle of pleasure alone. They compare the sexual act to a ritual or sacrament. This is because the person has to assume the responsibility of possibly bringing a new individual into birth. To procure progeny is the duty of every individual according to Hindu philosophy.

If the desire for sex is not fulfilled, it can result in physical or mental sickness. However, reckless, excessive, or perverted sexual activity results in loss of strength, weakening of immunity (Ojakshaya), disease, and death.

IMPORTANCE OF REPRODUCTIVE FLUIDS AND OJAS

Shukra or the reproductive fluid is the only tissue which leaves the body during the act of sexual intercourse. The function of this tissue is to give stability to the body. Hence loss of it results in loss of strength. Therefore, every attempt should be made to preserve all the tissues, particularly the reproductive as it is the most compact of them all and hence most difficult to replace.

Ojas is a very subtle material in the body and is considered as the purest form of all the tissues. It is responsible for body energy, brightness, strength, and immunity. It is comparable to Prana, the vital force, physical and mental strength. Excessive sexual activity results in loss of the reproductive fluid and Ojas. Therefore, restrained sexual activity is the key to physical as well as mental health.

RULES FOR SEXUAL ENJOYMENT

In the winter season (December–March), after taking Vajikaranas or aphrodisiac medicines, sex can be enjoyed according to one's desires; in the spring and autumn seasons (March–June and September–December), sex should only be enjoyed every fourth day; in summer (June–September), once every fifteen days is preferable.

Both partners must want to perform the act, and should be in good physical and mental health. A man should not engage in sex with a women during her menstrual period, or with one who is devoid of passion, unclean, too old, sick, or pregnant. For the woman, the man should similarly be healthy, clean, and passionate. Both partners, after enjoying the act, should preferably take a cool bath and drink cool water, milk, or wine. They should eat food containing natural sugars.

Individuals who do not regulate their sexual impulses are more prone to loss of strength, weak immune function, and various diseases owing to depletion of vitality. Those who regulate their sexual energy will have increased memory, power, intelligence, health, and longevity.

✳ ✳ ✳

REJUVENATION (RASAYANA)

Rasayana is a special type of treatment containing various methods of rejuvenation. It derives from "Rasa" and "Ayana." The literal meaning of Rasa is the essence of something. Anything ingested into the body in the form of food or medicine is first resynthesized into Rasa Dhatu, the basic plasma tissue. Ayana is the method by which Rasa is carried to all the body tissues for biochemical metamorphosis (Rasakriya). The concept of Rasayana is based on these two principles of conservation and transmutation of energy. Rasayana therapy strives to improve physical, mental, and moral qualities. It prevents old age, restores youthfulness, improves the complexion and the voice, increases physical strength and immunity. It strengthens memory and intelligence, gives happiness to oneself, and a life which is beneficial to others.

Every individual has a natural life span of a hundred years. The life span is nothing but the combined effect of reserve force of all organs, tissues, and systems. This reserve force is the combined effect of six components:

- Maternal influence
- Paternal influence
- Nutrition

- The subtle body
- The soul
- Congenital factors

If the optimum use of this reserve force is made, then one can achieve one's full life span. On the contrary, inordinate use of the sexual organs, improper food and rest, a reckless approach to the problems of life, and accumulation of stress and strain on the mind will consume the reserve force resulting in a shorter life span. Therefore individuals following ethical regimens will best achieve the benefits of Rasayana.

Preliminary Practices

In order to achieve the maximum benefit of Rasayana, the body must be made sensitive and receptive to assimilate the Rasayana medicine. Dirty clothes cannot be properly recolored unless the dirt is first removed. The same is the case with the human body.

Preliminary to Rasayana, Pancha Karma or the Five Purification Practices should be performed (see Chapter 9). Such practices aim at removing waste products and aggravated humors from the body. They also eliminate toxins (Ama) which are accumulated in the body due to disease as well as metabolic disorders and thereby make the body receptive to various rejuvenating methods.

An appropriate ethical regimen should also be followed. These are rules very similar to the Yama and Niyama practices of the Yoga system. The person who follows these rules achieves a steady and tranquil mind. This results in the withdrawal of the sense organs from disturbed activity and complete concentration in the Self, so that ultimately there is a minimum consumption of life energy. When this basal energy is converted into higher forms by the practice of Yoga, it becomes very beneficial for improving all brain functions.

How Rasayana Acts

The actions of Rasayana regimens are manifold:

- To increase body tissues
- To increase digestive power
- To increase the metabolic process at a tissue level or to improve endocrine gland function
- To remove waste products or to remove excess tissues in the body
- To increase the functional capacity of the brain

- To increase the strength and immunity of the body
- To destroy disease and establish homeostasis of energy, which prevents early aging

The effects of Rasayana therapy are better if the individual is young, has a healthy body and mind, possesses a good tolerance to physical and mental trauma, and has love for all creatures.

Types of Rasayana

There are two basic types of Rasayana therapy according to the place wherein the treatment is given:

- Allowing Movement or Ambulatory (Vatatapika)
- Requiring Inaction or Non-ambulatory (Kutipraveshika)

Rasayana therapies are also differentiated according to their purpose:

With specific purpose (Kamya):
- For improving longevity (Vayasthapana)
- For improving brain function (Medhya)
- For improving action of the tissues
- For improving action of the channel systems
- For improving action of the senses

To counteract a particular disease (Naimithik):
- Daily Rasayana (Ajasrik)
- Kutipraveshika

Of these above types, the non-ambulatory type of Rasayana is the most powerful and effective, and gives the maximum benefits of the therapy. A special type of building has to be constructed to do it, called a three-walled hut (Trigarbha Kuti). The idea behind the construction of such a building is that the person living inside it should not come into contact with the heat of the sun or dry wind, which take away vitality. If possible air conditioning and weatherproofing should be done. The room should have a stock of all required medicines and amenities necessary for daily life. The person who intends to undertake this special type of rejuvenation treatment should enter the building on an auspicious day after his body and mind have been purified by the necessary Pancha Karma practices and the correct ethical regimen. He should stay in this room for

·three months. During this period, he should avoid all contacts with the outside world and keep clear from all negative thoughts and emotions. To maintain tranquility of mind he should carry out meditation, Pranayama, and other necessary Yoga practices. During this Rasayana period he should eat only Rasayana substances, which have been prescribed by his Ayurvedic doctor. He should not take any other food.

Medicines

For Kutipraveshika Rasayana many formulas containing complex herbal drugs, called Divya Aushadhi, or "herbs having spiritual effects," are prescribed. Such are Brahma Rasayana, Chyavana Prash, and herbs like bhallataka, shilajit, and long pepper.

Ambulatory (Vatatapika)

This type of Rasayana can be done while engaged in daily activities. Although of less benefit than the previous method, it is suitable for everyone. However, one should not consume excess oily, fatty, or spicy food. A sensate life style and the drinking of alcohol should be totally given up. All the Rasayana substances mentioned can be used in this type of treatment.

General Rasayanas

For promoting longevity, retarding the aging process, and prolonging youthfulness, medicines like guduchi are advised. These can be taken like food suppliments as general rasayanas.

For increasing the qualitative and quantitative functional capacity of the brain, herbs which provide nutrition to the brain centers are indicated. They help increase intelligence, memory, and quick comprehension. Herbs like calamus, shankhapushpi, jatamansi, brahmi, and mandukaparni are some of the best rejuvenatives for the brain (Medhya Rasayanas). They accelerate the development of the faculties of the higher brain centers.

For specific tissues, certain herbs and foods function as Rasayanas. Some of these are:

Plasma (Rasa)	Draksha, shatavari, dates
Blood (Rakta)	Amalaki, lauhadi rasayana, bhringaraj, suvarna makshika
Muscle (Mamsa)	Masha, ashwagandha, bala, nux vomica, silver bhasma
Fat (Meda)	Guggul, shilajit, haritaki, guduchi, garlic

Bone (Asthi)	Shukti (mother of pearl) bhasma, prawal (coral) bhasma, kukkutanda bhasma, mrigashringa bhasma, vamsharochan, prishnaparni
Nerve (Majja)	Calamus, gotu kola, shankhapushpi, loha bhasma, gold bhasma, makaradhwaja
Reproductive (Shukra)	Kapikacchu, vidarikanda, shatavari, ashwagandha, ghee and milk from the cow

Just as for the tissues, different herbs and foods function as Rasayanas for the different channel-systems. The Rasayanas for the other channel-systems are the same as those for their respective tissues.

Respiratory	Chyavan Prash, Vardhaman pippali (long pepper), Vardhaman marich (black pepper)
Digestive	Long pepper, bhallataka, haritaki, Suvarna Parpati
Water	Fresh ginger, cyperus, cardamom
Urinary	Punarnava, gokshura
Excretory	Kutaj, vidanga, Triphala
Sweat	Basil, nux vomica, datura

Vardhaman Rasayana is a special method by which tissues in the body are saturated with a particular medicine by unit increase and unit decrease method.

For Vardhaman Pippali, take one-half cup of water and one-half cup of milk, add one long pepper (pippali) on the first day, boil until the water evaporates, and drink the milk. On the second and successive days, add one additional pippali until the total amount reaches the number of seven, nine, or eleven. Then reduce the amount taken each day by one until the amount of one long pepper is again reached. This cycle should be repeated for three months. For Vardhaman Marich (black pepper), start with two black pepper corns and increase the amount by two. Go up to sixteen, eighteen, or twenty pepper corns and gradually reduce the amount again to two, also for a three month period. This is a slow method of rebuilding the lung tissue, which thereby does not damage the lungs and increases their energy in a way that persists for a long period of time.

For the senses and other organs:

Eye	Triphala, licorice, shatavari
Nose	Nasya of Anu Tail
Skin	Tuvarak, catechu, bakuchi
Brain	Gotu kola, calamus
Heart	Guggul, elecampane, gold bhasma
Neuro-Muscular System	Bala, nagbala, garlic, guggul

Rasayana According to Constitution

For Vata	Bala, ashwagandha
For Pitta	Amalaki, shatavari, guduchi
For Kapha	Bhallataka, guggul, long pepper, garlic

THE USE OF APHRODISIACS (VAJIKARANA)

Charaka has affirmed that every human being possesses three basic innate urges or drives — the instinct for self-preservation, the instinct to gain wealth, and the instinct for self-realization. The desire to have children is the attempt to fulfill the first of these three desires, that of preserving life. Although the science of Vajikarana attempts to increase sexual power, its real aim is genetic improvement. It has been clearly stated that those who are unable to control their sexual urge should not use these medicines. This method should be adopted after the person attains the age of puberty and when hormones and secondary sex characteristics have developed. It should not be used before the age of sixteen and after the age of seventy.

Like Rasayana, purification of body and mind are essential for achieving the maximum benefits of Vajikarana. For purification of the body, Charaka has suggested the use of Niruha and Yapana Basti.

DIFFERENCES BETWEEN RASAYANA AND VAJIKARANA

Rasayana	Vajikarana
Advisable for male and female	Needed mainly by men (Woman herself is the best Vajikarana)
Useful in all age groups	Should not be used before sixteen or after seventy
Can be used to eradicate certain diseases	Not useful to eradicate diseases

Rasayana	Vajikarana
Sexual contact to be avoided	Sexual enjoyment with restraint
Aim is to prepare healthy self-realization	Aim is to fulfill urge to preserve life through good progeny
Medicines are composed of all five elements	Predominantly earth and water elements

Vajikarana Medicines

In many Vajikarana preparations, the eggs of different birds, the flesh of various animals (including birds and fish) and their testicles have been used, as well as cow's milk, honey, ghee, and sugar. Traditional Chinese medicine uses similar items in the same way. Again the yogic precautions against meat and eggs should be taken into consideration. Similarly the following herbs are useful:

Cane sugar, shatavari, ashwagandha, licorice, garlic, saffron, masha, bala, mahabala, vidarikanda, kapikacchu, gokshura, meda, kokilaksha, and kakoli

PART II

METHODS
OF AYURVEDIC TREATMENT

6
THE AYURVEDIC SCIENCE
OF HEALING SUBSTANCES

Every system of medicine uses various substances in healing. Each has its theory whereby these medicines are employed. Ayurveda possesses one of the most sophisticated of such theories. The Ayurvedic science of medicinal substances is called Dravyaguna. It refers to substances (Dravya), their properties (Guna), and their actions (Karma). It deals with all the aspects of herbal and mineral medicines such as identification, usage, dosage, and methods of processing both for the promotion of health and treatment of disease.

Ayurveda accepts the law of uniformity in nature. According to this, medicinal substances and living bodies are similar in composition, both being products of the same cosmic forces. Hence herbs and drugs influence the body according to their nature and attributes. Substances of opposite attributes can be used to correct conditions of imbalance within the body.

BRANCHES

AYURVEDIC PHARMACOGNOSY, the identification of medicinal substances, knowledge of their name and form. This branch deals with various classifications of herbs and their morphological character, a botanical approach.

AYURVEDIC PHARMACOLOGY, the science of the properties and actions of medicines. This classifies medicines according to their energetics as defined by Ayurveda.

AYURVEDIC PHARMACEUTICS, the Ayurvedic science of preparing medicines including decoctions, powders, pills, tablets, herbal wines, etc. It also deals with the collection and storage of drugs.

AYURVEDIC THERAPEUTICS, the science of employing medicines Ayurvedically. It deals with the uses of medicines in various diseases, including dosage, time of ingestion and mediums for taking them, as well as the sites in the body at which they are absorbed.

Each thing in the universe is a substance, as defined by the properties and actions it possesses. All substances are composed of different degrees of the five great elements. As the human body is also composed of the same elements, all substances can be used as medicines when they are applied with a definite purpose and rationale to correct bodily imbalances.

AYURVEDIC CLASSIFICATION OF MEDICINES
According to Use
This is as food (ahara), poison (visha), or herb (aushadha).

Herbs may be strong in potency like bhallataka (marking nut), which can cause severe allergic reactions, or aconite, which is poisonous; they may be medium in potency, which includes most herbs of bitter, pungent, or astringent tastes; or they may be mild in potency and safe for long-term usage, like amalaki, marshmallow, and most tonic and nutritive herbs.

According to Energetics
This is by elemental constituents, taste (Rasa), potency (Virya), post-digestive effect (Vipaka), and special action (Prabhava), which is explained below.

According to Source of Derivation
These are twofold as organic (chetana) and inorganic (achetana). Organic substances derive from either animals or plants. Animal sources are mammals (jayajuya, born from the womb), birds and fishes (andaja, born from eggs), insects (svedaja, born from moisture), and worms (udbhijja, born from the earth). Plant sources are large trees with fruit but no apparent flowers (vanaspati), like tropical fig trees; medium trees with both fruits and flowers (vriksha), like mango or citrus; shrubs and small plants (virudha); herbaceous plants and grasses (oshadhi).

According to Action on the Doshas
Herbs may either pacify (shamana), purify (shodhana), aggravate (kopana), or maintain (swasthahita) the Doshas.

THE FIFTY THERAPEUTIC ACTIONS
Charaka has defined fifty groups of herbs according to their therapeutic action. Each group containing ten herbs is called a "Mahakashaya." By the application of the method of induction, taking common character-

istics into account, other similar herbs can be incorporated into these groups. These groups are as follows:

1. VITALIZING AGENTS (Jivaniya), help protect one's life and promote longevity like licorice or mung beans

2. BULK-PROMOTING AGENTS (Brimhaniya), increase bodily weight and promote formation of new tissues as in the case of ashwagandha, bala, and marshmallow

3. REDUCING AGENTS (Lekhaniya), reduce fat or other accumulations; examples: cyperus, turmeric, black pepper, or barberry

4. ACCUMULATION-BREAKING AGENTS (Bhedaniya), break down stronger accumulations like gall or kidney stones; chitrak, kutaj, pashana bheda

5. HEALING AGENTS (Sandhaniya), promote the healing of wounds or cuts; manjishta, turmeric, aloe gel, bayberry

6. DIGESTIVE STIMULANTS (Dipaniya), enkindle the digestive fire (Agni); dry ginger, black pepper, long pepper, chitrak

7. TONICS (Balya), strength-giving herbs; bala, ashwagandha, shatavari, ginseng

8. COMPLEXION-IMPROVING AGENTS (Varnya); sandalwood, turmeric, lotus root, manjishtha

9. BENEFICIAL FOR THE THROAT (Kanthya), for soothing sore throat and improving the voice; raisins, vidari, bayberry, haritaki, licorice

10. HEART TONICS (Hridya); pomegranate fruit, arjuna, mango, hawthorne berries

11. ANTI-SATURATIVE (Triptighna), relieve false sense of contentment, as under excess Kapha; ginger, guduchi, calamus

12. ANTI-HEMORRHOIDAL (Arsoghna); kutaj, ginger, haritaki, calamus

13. ANTI-DERMATOSIS (Kusthaghna), reduce skin inflammations; catechu, turmeric, haritaki, amalaki

14. ANTI-PRURITIC (Kandughna), relieve itching on the skin; neem bark, barberry, licorice

15. ANTHELMINTIC (Krimighna), destroy parasites; vidanga, betel nuts, pumpkin seeds

16. ANTI-TOXIN (Vishaghna), counter poisons; shirisha, turmeric, sandalwood

17. LACTOGOGUES (Stanya-janana), promote secretion of breast milk; shatavari, fennel, dill

18. LACTODEPURANTS (Stanya-shodhana), purify breast milk; guduchi, ginger, dandelion

19. SPERMOGENIC (Shukra-janana), increase sperm count; vidari, ashwagandha, shatavari, lotus seeds

20. PURIFY SPERM (Shukra-shodhana); kushta, bayberry, vetivert

21. OLEATING ADJUNCTIVE (Snehopaga), help facilitate absorption of oils; raisins, licorice, vidari

22. ADJUNCTS TO SWEATING THERAPY (Swedopaga), allow for easier sweating (not diaphoretics or sweat-inducing however); castor root, barley, sesame, black gram, mung beans

23. ADJUNCTS TO EMESIS (Vamanopaga), aid in the process of vomiting; honey, licorice

24. ADJUNCTS TO PURGATION (Virecanopaga), usually laxative in nature; raisins, prunes, haritaki, amalaki

25. ADJUNCTS TO DECOCTION ENEMAS (Asthapanopaga), help cleanse Vata from the colon; bilwa, pippali, calamus, licorice

26. ADJUNCTIVES TO OILY ENEMAS (Anuvasanopaga), help calm Vata in the colon; fennel, gokshura, bilwa

27. ADJUNCTIVES TO CLEANSING NASAL THERAPY (Shirovirecanopaga), help remove Kapha from above the neck; black pepper, long pepper, mustard

28. ANTI-EMETICS (Chardini-nigrahana), stop vomiting; cardamom, fresh ginger, vetivert, puffed rice

29. THIRST-RELIEVING (Trishna-nigrahana); sandalwood, coriander, ginger (for thirst owing to Kapha)

30. STOP HICCUPS (Hikka-nigrahana); elecampane, haritaki, long pepper

31. GIVE FORM TO THE FECES (Purisha-samgraniya); astringents like lodhra, pomegranate husks, some forms of clay

32. GIVE COLOR TO THE STOOL (Purisha-virajiniya); catechu, lotus root, licorice, sesame seed

33. ANTI-DIURETICS (Mutra-sangrahniya), stop excessive urination; bhallataka, rose hips

34. GIVE COLOR TO THE URINE (Mutra-virajinya); lotus seed, lotus root, licorice

35. DIURETICS (Mutra-virecaniya), promote urination; gokshura, punarnava, coriander, lemon grass

36. STOP COUGH (Kasahara), anti-tussive; phyllanthus, haritaki, raisins, sumach

37. COUNTER ASTHMA (Shwasahara), stop wheezing, ease breathing; elecampane, cardamom, basil

38. RELIEVE EDEMA AND SWELLING (Shotahara); mainly diuretics and astringents like bilwa and gokshura

39. FEBRIFUGE (Jwarahara), relieve fevers; Draksha, manjishta, Triphala, raw sugar, bitters generally

40. RELIEVE FATIGUE (Shramahara), as from overexposure to heat; dates, pomegranate juice, sugar cane, raisins

41. RELIEVE BURNING SENSATION ON THE SKIN (Daha-prashamana); sandalwood, vetivert, lotus leaf, raw sugar

42. RELIEVE COLD SENSATION ON THE SKIN (Shita-prashamana); valerian, agaru, calamus, long pepper, ginger, coriander

43. RELIEVE SKIN RASHES (Udarda-prashamana), as for urticaria; catechu, arjuna

44. RELIEVE BODY ACHE (Angamarda-prashama), to cure malaise, as from fever or flu; sandalwood, cardamom, mint, camphor

45. RELIEVE COLIC PAIN (Shula-prashamana), analgesic and anti-spasmodic for smooth muscle; ajwan, fennel, dill, ginger, long pepper

46. STOPPING BLEEDING (Shonita-sthapana), hemostatic; licorice, lodhra, honey, red clay, agrimony

47. RELIEVE PAIN (Vedana-sthapana) sedatives for nerve pain; valerian, jatamansi, shirisha, bayberry

48. RESTORE CONSCIOUSNESS (Samjña-stapana), as from coma or delirium; gotu kola (brahmi), calamus, asafoetida, camphor

49. PROMOTE REPRODUCTION (Praja-sthapana), cure sterility, remove obstructions in genital tract; amalaki, haritaki, gotu kola (brahmi), katuka

50. PROMOTE LONGEVITY (Vaya-sthapana), rejuvenative; guduchi sattva, haritaki, gotu kola, shatavari, amalaki

COMMON GROUPS OF HERBS

The following are some common herbal formulas used in Ayurveda either by themselves or as part of greater formulas.

GROUPS	CONSTITUENTS
Triphala The three fruits: laxative, rejuvenative	Haritaki, bibhitaka, amalaki
Trikatu The three spices: stimulant, digestive	Dry ginger, long pepper, black pepper
Trijata Carminative, anti-emetic	Cinnamon, cardamom, cinnamon leaf
Chaturjata Carminative, appetizer	Trijata and nagakeshar
Trimada Clears consciousness, opens channels, removes obstructions	Vidanga, cyperus, chitrak
Chaturbija The four seeds: carminative, stimulant	Fenugreek, watercress, kalajaji, yavani
Pañchakola Digestive, stimulant	Long pepper (pippali), pippali root, chavya, chitrak, dry ginger
Pañchavalkala The five barks: astringent, anti-styptic, anti-diuretic, hemostatic	Barks of nyagrodha, udumbara, ashwattha, plaksha, parisha
Pañchapallava Astringent, anti-diarrhea, for diabetes	Mango, jambu, kapittha, citron, bilwa
Trinapañchamula Increase urination, for urinary tract stones	Kusha, kasa, nala, darbha, sugar cane

Pañchatikta
  The five bitters: antipyretic,
    febrifuge, alterative

Vasa, guduchi, neem, kantakari,
patola

Brihat Pañchamula
  The greater five roots: alleviates Vata

Bilwa, patala, agnimantha,
syonaka, sambhari

Laghu Pañchamula
  The lesser five roots: alleviates Vata

Shalaparni, prishniparni,
kantakari, gokshura, brihati

Dashamula
  The ten roots: alleviates Vata, good
  for basty (enema therapy)

Combines Brihat and Laghu
Panchamula

THE FIVE GREAT ELEMENTS IN HERBS

The five great elements are responsible for the formation of the universe as well as man. Their properties and actions are as follows:

Earth	Smell	Sweet, slightly astringent Promotes growth, weight gain, compactness of tissues, stability, strength, downward flow of Prana (purgation)
Water	Taste	All tastes, mainly sweet Cold, wet, slow, heavy, mobile, liquid, soft, sticky Moistening, oleating, binding, holding in solution, pleasing
Fire	Sight	Pungent, slightly sour and salty Hot, sharp, subtle, rough, hard, light, clear Warming, digestive stimulant, gives luster, improves complexion, gives illumination, causes tearing, burning, moving upwards (emetic, expectorant)
Air	Touch	Astringent, slightly bitter Subtle, hard, cold, light, clear Cleansing, giving lightness, roughening, agitating
Ether	Sound	No taste Loosening, subtle, soft, penetrating, discriminating Softening, increasing porousness, opening channels, giving lightness

The Five Elements in Nature

All earthy substances are hard, solid, and dense, or soft, moldable, and shapeful in character. They give smell or fragrance only when rendered to powder form. All watery substances have a certain amount of fluid that can be judged by the juice or watery content within them. Fire-dominant substances are easy to crush, they emit a strong odor and are of bright color. A substance with dusky colors and having thin, hard, patchy architecture as well as a rough texture is of an air-dominant. Ether-dominant substances are easy to compress and disintegrate but do not exhibit color or odor.

∗ ∗ ∗

THE ENERGETICS OF HEALING SUBSTANCES: RASA-VIRYA-VIPAKA-PRABHAVA

Taste (Rasa)

The taste of a substance, which can be perceived by the tongue, is known as Rasa. Each taste (Rasa) indicates the preponderance of two of the five primordial elements. It is according to the similarity between the preponderant elements in the herbs or the diet on one hand, and the Doshas on the other, that the herbs and diet are selected and used.

Taste and Aftertaste

Each substance is composed of all five elements. Hence it is impossible to find a substance having only one Rasa. When a substance is called sour, this does not exclude the other tastes. It only means that the sour taste is predominant, while the others are unmanifest.

Hence Rasa is manifest, stable in the dry state and is perceived at first, while aftertaste (Anurasa) is unstable in the dry state, and perceived in the fresh state after the Rasa.

FORMATION OF THE RASAS FROM THE ELEMENTS

Elements	Rasas
Ether + Air	Tikta – Bitter
Air + Fire	Katu – Pungent
Fire + Water	Lavana – Saline, salty
Water + Earth	Madhura – Sweet, plain taste
Earth + Fire	Amla – Sour
Earth + Air	Kashaya – Astringent

We have already seen that for building up body tissues, earth and water constitutents are most useful. Hence sweet, sour, and astringent Rasas only are good for this purpose. On the other hand, substances having bitter, pungent, and salty tastes are useful for reducing the body tissues.

Inference of Taste from Plant Characteristics

Plants exhibiting fully developed features including roots, stem, branches, foliage, covered seeds, and efflorescence usually possess a pleasant or sweet taste and are useful for nourishment. This is because sweet taste derives from earth and water.

Plants that are long living, bulky, and hard usually have an astringent taste, as this taste derives from earth and air. Although sour taste derives from earth and fire, plants yielding sour taste contain less bulk and need support to stand.

As the pungent taste is formed by fire and air, these plants do not have hard or well-formed characteristics, nor do they contain any juice in them. But they usually have bright colored flowers and often have aromatic volatile oils. There are very few plants that have a salty taste, as it is the combination of fire and water. Pure bitter taste is formed by ether and air; hence plants yielding only bitter taste are light and lacking in bulk.

Classification of the Tastes

The six tastes are classified into two groups according to the Agni-Soma concept.

FIERY (Agneya) tastes — Pungent (Katu), Sour (Amla) and Salty (Lavana) increase the digestive power and Pitta.

WATERY (Saumya) tastes — Sweet (Madhura), Bitter (Tikta) and Astringent (Kashaya) decrease Pitta.

TASTE	QUALITY (GUNA) RELATION
Sweet	Damp, cold, heavy
Sour	Damp, hot, light
Saline	Damp, hot, heavy
Pungent	Dry, hot, light
Bitter	Dry, cold, light
Astringent	Dry, cold, heavy

By these three sets of qualities we can discriminate the differences between the six tastes. Heavy means heavy for digestion; light means easy for digestion.

Relation of Tastes and Humors

We have observed that the six tastes represent six different combinations of the five great elements and their resultant activity. As sweet taste is produced by the combination of earth and water, for example, therefore it will increase the earthy and watery components of the body, Kapha. Similarly, it will decrease the opposite components of air and fire elements, Pitta and Vata. Hence sweet, sour, and salty tastes increase Kapha, while pungent, bitter, and astringent tastes reduce it. Conversely, sweet, sour, and salty tastes decrease Vata while pungent, bitter, and astringent increase it. Pungent, sour, and salty increase Pitta, while bitter, astringent, and sweet reduce it. The six tastes thereby increase or decrease the Doshas in a regular manner. But to do this the herb or food cannot go directly into the tissues as such. It must first pass through the digestive process. This aspect is dealt with under post-digestive effect.

SYSTEMIC ACTION OF TASTES

SWEET TASTE — is homologous with the body from birth. It increases body nutrient fluid, blood, muscle, fat, bone, nerve tissue, and semen. It prolongs life, clarifies the sense organs, imparts vigor and complexion, decreases Pitta, Vata, and toxins in the body. It has a beneficial influence on the skin, hair, voice, and strength. It promotes cheerfulness, vitality, and satisfaction. It increases body tissues and makes the body firm. It is cold, slightly oily, and heavy for digestion. Excess use of the sweet taste produces obesity, lethargy, heaviness, loss of appetite, dyspnea, cough, cold, constipation, vomiting, and other diseases of Kapha.

SOUR TASTE — increases the pleasure of eating, stimulates digestive power, builds up body tissues, enlightens the mind, stabilizes the sense functions, promotes strength, and regulates peristalsis, and the movements of Vata. It promotes nutrition of the heart and causes salivation. It conducts the food downward in the gastro-inestinal tract, moistens it, and aids in its proper digestion. It is light, hot, and oily in character. Excessive use produces thirst, dissolves Kapha, increases Pitta, vitiates blood, causes sloughing of muscles, renders the body tissue loose, and produces edema in emaciated persons.

SALTY TASTE — helps digestion, removes obstructions in the channels, is laxative, and diminishes Vata, stiffness, and accumulations. It overpowers the other tastes, increases secretions in the mouth. It liquefies mucus, gives relish to the food, is neither very heavy nor oily and is hot. Excessive use increases Pitta, vitiates the blood, and provokes thirst. It causes corrosion of the flesh, aggravates dermal lesions and toxins in the body, destroys virility, impairs the function of the nervous system, induces premature wrinkles on the skin, grey hair, and baldness.

PUNGENT TASTE — purifies the mouth, stimulates digestion, causes running of the nose and watering of mouth and eyes, and sharpens the sense organs. It helps to reduce edema and obesity, and removes excess oiliness in the body. It eliminates excretory matter, imparts relish to food, and decreases itching. It is vermicidal, causes lacerations in flesh, breaks accumulations of the blood, removes obstructions, dilates the channels, and decreases Kapha. It is light, hot, and dry in character. Excess use destroys virility and gives rise to emaciation. It produces fainting, choking, giddiness, and burning sensations. It produces heat in the body, diminishes strength, and produces thirst.

BITTER TASTE — although it produces an unpleasant taste in the mouth, it has an appetizing action. It helps to get rid of poisons, is vermicidal, relieves burning sensation, itching, thirst, and diseases of the skin. It imparts firmness to skin and flesh. It has an anti-febrile quality and digestive action, aiding in reducing obesity. It takes out extra water from lymph, sweat, urine, feces, bile, and mucus. It is dry, cold, and light in character. Excessive use produces dryness, loss of strength, and generates many Vata diseases.

ASTRINGENT TASTE — decreases Kapha, increases Vata, and has styptic and healing properties. It purifies the blood, removes an excess of watery waste products from the body, and is dry and cold in character. Excessive use produces dryness in the mouth and skin. It constricts the channels, obstructs speech, and produces gas in the stomach and intestines. It inhibits the excretion of feces, urine, and sweat, and produces many Vata diseases.

ACTION OF TASTES
On Tissues

Two tastes increase bodily tissues: sweet taste increases all bodily tissues, while sour taste increases all except reproductive tissue. The other four tastes (salty, pungent, bitter and astringent) decrease bodily tissues.

On Waste Materials

The earth and water dominant group (sweet, sour, and salty tastes) facilitate the movement of waste materials, are laxative, carminative, and increase urination. The air dominant group (pungent, bitter, and astringent tastes) inhibit the waste materials, cause flatulence or constipation, and are drying.

On Agni (The Digestive Fire)

Fiery (Agneya) tastes (pungent, sour, and salty) increase Agni, promote appetite, and burn Ama or toxins. Bitter taste, although of the watery (Saumya) group stimulates Agni by promoting Samana Vayu. Sweet and astringent tastes decrease Agni.

On the Channel Systems

Channel cleansing (Srotoshodhana) — Pungent taste, due to air and fire constituents, absorbs fluid and expels obstructive material in the channels. Bitter taste has the same qualities. In addition, because of its subtle quality, bitter taste permeates even to the minutest channels. Salty taste liquefies solids and expels them due to its penetrating quality. Sweet, sour, and astringent tastes have no such effect; they act to clog or block the channels.

POST-DIGESTIVE EFFECT (VIPAKA)

When an herb or food is ingested, it is acted upon by the digestive fire. During this process, the six tastes (Rasas) are resynthesized into the three post-digestive effects (Vipakas). Even though post-digestive effect is explained in the terminology of the tastes — sweet (Madhura) Vipaka, sour (Amla) Vipaka, and pungent (Katu) Vipaka — they cannot be identified by the tongue or sense of taste. Vipaka is also called "isthapaka," as opposed to Avasthapaka or Prapaka, which is formed during the stages of digestion. Avasthapaka is the transient phase of digestion while Vipaka is the final transformation of ingested material.

Post-digestive Effect

Post-digestive effect is inferred from the final action of the ingested food or medicine. As there are two main effects, namely building or anabolic (Brimhana) and reducing or catabolic (Langhana), post-digestive effect is of two types only — heavy (building) and light (reducing). This is the classification of Sushruta according to the effect of Vipaka on the tissues. The classification of post-digestive effect by Charaka is according to its effect on the Doshas. He classifies Vipaka into three types — sweet, sour,and pungent. Out of these three, sweet is the same as heavy, while sour and pungent are included under light.

Post-digestive effect is seen mainly in the field of Apana Vayu; on discharges like urine, feces, semen, the menstrual discharge, and the fetus. Also its action can be grouped under anabolic and catabolic results.

TASTE	POST-DIGESTIVE EFFECT	ACTION
Sweet Saline	Sweet	Promotes Kapha, smoothly eliminates feces and urine, increases reproductive fluids
Sour	Sour	Promotes Pitta, smoothly eliminates feces and urine, diminishes reproductive fluids
Pungent Bitter Astringent	Pungent	Promotes Vata, suppresses feces and urine, diminishes reproductive fluids

ENERGY OF HERBS (VIRYA)

Virya is the potency by which the action of a substance takes place. It literally means "vigor." Hence herbs devoid of Virya will be inactive. It is also seen that often an herb or drug loses its potency after a certain amount of time. This can be owing to the effect of time or because of improper processing or storage. The most active attribute in a substance is called Virya. Out of the twenty primary attributes only eight have the potential to become Virya. They are light and heavy, cold and hot, unctuous and rough, and soft and sharp. Sushruta replaces light and heavy with clear and cloudy, probably because he mentions them as two types of post-digestive effects.

However, Virya has ultimately been grouped into two types only. Based on the concept of Agni and Soma, Virya is classified as either hot or cold. Hence Ayurveda speaks of the energy of substances as primarily heating or cooling, recognizing within this classification differences of degrees.

ACTIONS OF ENERGY (VIRYA)

Type	Action on Doshas	General Effect
Hot	Pacifies Kapha and Vata, Aggravates Pitta	Helps digestion, causes hot sensation, thirst, diaphoresis
Cold	Pacifies Pitta, Aggravates Kapha and Vata	Cooling, exhilarant, moistening, enlivening, increases semen

Relation with Taste and Post-digestive Effect

Substances having sweet taste and post-digestive effect are generally cooling in energy (Shita Virya); while those having sour and pungent tastes and post-digestive effects are most often heating (Ushna Virya). Usually Virya (energy) dominates Rasa (taste) and Vipaka (post-digestive action).

SPECIAL POTENCY (PRABHAVA)

The special or specific potency of an herb is called Prabhava. It is observed when two drugs having similar taste, energy, and post-digestive effect differ in action. Although it is very difficult to explain the exact nature of Prabhava, it may be due either to specific elemental combinations or to specificity in the site of an herb's action (for example, the cardiotonic activity of arjuna).

Types of Prabhava

ANTI-TOXIC — some plants like shirisha show this type of Prabhava

BACTERICIDAL — some plants like guggul, myrrh, or garlic have this

PURGATIVES — some bitters have this Prabhava

GHEE AND MILK — both are sweet in Rasa and Vipaka and cold in potency, but ghee increases Agni and milk does not

ACTION OF MEDICINAL SUBSTANCES

Medicinal action or karma is that which causes combination or separation, unification or division. In the context of the Ayurvedic science of medicinal substances it is related to the action of an herb on the humors, tissues, waste materials, systems, and organs of the body. All medicinal substances, being external forms of the five elements, are first converted into five element forms within the body. Then they can influence respective humors, tissues, waste materials, and systems. This action can be localized or systemic, direct or indirect.

CLASSIFICATION OF HERBAL ACTIONS

By Therapies

PURIFICATION (Shodhana) is of five types:
- Emesis (Vamana)
- Purgation (Virechana)
- Blood purification (Raktamokshana)

- Oil containing enema (Anuvasana)
- Decoction enema (Asthapana).

PALLIATION (Shamana) is of two types:
- Building (Brimhana) which includes oleation (Snehana) and astringent action (Stambhana)
- Reducing (Langhana) which includes drying (Rukshana) and sudation (Swedana).

By Humors, Tissues, and Waste-Materials Effected

Therapies can be classified according to their effect on the Doshas, tissues, and waste-materials.

ACTION ON DOSHAS

Vata-reducing	Sesame oil
Pitta-reducing	Ghee
Kapha-reducing	Honey
Vata-aggravating	Beans
Pitta-aggravating	Mustard
Kapha-aggravating	Cheese

ACTION ON TISSUES

Fat-reducing	Guggul, myrrh
Blood-cleansing	Turmeric, red clover
Muscle-relaxing	Valerian

ACTION ON WASTE MATERIALS

Increasing the stool	Barley, psyllium
Promoting sweat	Ginger, cinnamon, basil
Promoting urination	Punarnava, gokshura

BY CHANNEL SYSTEMS AFFECTED
DIGESTIVE SYSTEM

Improving taste (Rochana)	Citrus fruits
Digestive stimulants (Dipana)	Asafoetida
Digestive agents (Pachana)	Dry Ginger

Gastric irritant (Vidahi)	Chili
Astringent (Vishtambhi)	Jack fruit
Emetic (Vamana)	Emetic Nut, lobelia
Anti-emetic (Chardi Nigraha)	Cardamom

EXCRETORY SYSTEM

Purgative (Virechana)	Castor oil, trivrit
Anti-diarrhea	Kutaj, alum
Asthapana (corrective enemas)	Dashamula
Anuvasana (medicated oil enemas)	Sesame oil
Anthelmintic (Krimighna)	Vidanga

RESPIRATORY SYSTEM

Anti-cough (Kasahara)	Sumach
Anti-asthma (Shwasahara)	Vasa, mullein
Heart tonic (Hridya)	Arjuna

CIRCULATORY SYSTEM

Alterative (Rakta Prasadana)	Nagkeshar

SEBACEOUS SYSTEM

Promote sweating (Swedana)	Nagkeshar

* * *

PRIME ATTRIBUTES (GUNA)

Ayurveda describes forty-one prime attributes (Gunas). These are in four groups:

- The twenty qualities of substances (Gurvadi)
- The ten qualities of application (Paradi)
- The five special qualities (Vishishtha)
- The six psychological qualities (Adhyatmika)

The term Guna mean quality, mode, or property. Out of these only the twenty attributes are used in pharmacology. These twenty properties are placed in two groups of ten; as qualities essential for tissue gain or those responsible for tissue loss. The factors which promote new cellular units are termed Samanya or homologous. The factors which promote destruction of tissues, are called Vishesha or heterologous.

The Twenty Attributes (Gurvadi Guna)

These are also referred to as bodily properties (Sharira Gunas) as they are found in body tissue as well as in the substances which influence them. They are physical as well as pharmacological in action.

THE TWENTY ATTRIBUTES AND THEIR ACTIONS

GUNA	COMPOSITION*	ACTION
Heavy (Guru)	E–W	Building (Brimhana)
Light (Laghu)	F–A–Eth	Reducing (Langhana)
Cold (Shita)	W	Cooling (Stambhana)
Hot (Ushna)	F	Heating (Swedana)
Wet (Snigdha)	W	Moistening (Kledana)
Dry (Ruksha)	E–F–A	Absorbing (Shoshana)
Dull (Manda)	E–W	Slowing-Pacifying (Shamana)
Sharp (Tikshna)	F	Penetrating-Purifying (Shodhana)
Firm (Sthira)	E	Stabilizing (Dharana)
Mobile (Sara)	A	Stimulating (Prerana)
Smooth (Mridu)	W–Eth	Loosening (Shlathana)
Hard (Kathina)	E	Hardening (Dridhikarana)
Clear (Vishada)	E–F–A–Eth	Cleansing (Kshalana)
Sticky (Picchhila)	W	Adhering (Lepana)
Soft (Shalkshna)	W–E	Healing (Ropana)
Rough (Khara)	A	Scraping (Lekhana)
Subtle (Sukshma)	A	Pervading (Vivarana)
Gross (Sthula)	E	Covering (Samvarana)
Dense (Sandra)	E–W	Solidifying (Prasadana)
Fluid (Drava)	W	Liquefying (Vilodana)

*E=Earth, W=Water, F=Fire, A=Air, Eth=Ether

(See also Qualities of Food for more information on these attributes)

The Ten Qualities of Application (Paradi Gunas)

These are widely used in treatment, pharmacy, etc. and indicate the factors for the right applications of medicines.

Para	Preferable, superior
Apara	Not preferable, inferior
Yukti	Rationale, method
Samkhya	Enumeration
Samyoga	Combination
Vibhaga	Division
Prithaktva	Separateness
Parimana	Weights and measures
Samskara	Processing
Abhyasa	Repeated use

We must consider whether the medicines we are using are of superior or inferior power, what is the rationale or strategy behind their usage, the number of their applications, whether they are combined with other substances or divided up into smaller parts, whether they are employed separately or together, in what amounts, according to what processing, and in what frequency.

The Five Special Qualities (Vishishtha Gunas)

These are the most basic qualities, those that relate to the five senses. They are sound, touch, sight, taste, and smell (shabda, sparsha, rupa, rasa, gandha). These are the five Tanmatras that underlie all perceptible phenomena in the universe. We must consider the impressions (tanmatras) we are receiving in all of our activities in life. These can enhance or counteract the effect of treatment.

The Six Psychological Qualities (Adhyatmika Gunas)

These are the main qualities at work in the mind: Buddhi, intellect or judgment; Iccha, desire; Dwesha, aversion; Sukha, pleasure; Duhkha, pain; Prayatna, effort or volition. Each mental state involves one of these qualities. First we must ascertain (Buddhi) the nature of a condition; this leads to attraction (Iccha) to what we have decided is good and repulsion (Dwesha) to what we think is bad. The gaining of what we think is good gives rise to pleasure (Sukha), while experiencing what we think is bad causes pain (Duhkha). This gives rise to effort or action (Prayatna) to hold on to what gives happiness and to avoid what causes suffering.

According to Yoga and Ayurveda we must seek out those things that give enduring happiness, as opposed to merely following those which give temporary pleasure. Hence it is important that we learn to ascertain the inner truth of things. This right judgment is the basis of right effort. No one wants pain, but in wrongly seeking lasting happiness in temporary pleasure, the mind gets confused and the result is disease.

In treatment we must consider the psychological qualities of the patient and how to guide them through right judgment to right action. Similarly the doctor must also adequately judge the nature of a condition to lead to right action to improve the condition and to alleviate pain.

AYURVEDIC MEDICINES

Charaka has given an excellent definition of the ideal medicine, while classifying substances into three groups — food, medicine, and poison.

Substances which are mainly useful for tissue building like wheat, rice, and milk are food substances. Substances which, after entering the body, get eliminated through the gastro-intestinal tract within a specified period after their corrective role is over are medicines. This includes most herbs, which affect bodily processes, like the increased sweating that comes through hot herbs like ginger, but which do not function as foods.

While poisons are not homologous for the formation of new tissues, they stick to different tissues in the body and cause many harmful effects. Accumulation of such substances decreases the functional capability of the entire body, as we are witnessing with the various forms of heavy metal toxicity in our modern polluted environment.

There is some overlap between these categories. Foods have some medicinal effects, like the action of barley to increase urination. Some herbs, tonics like ashwagandha, have tissue building action like foods. Poisons can have some limited medicinal action. By this theory all chemical drugs are poisons and must have some side-effects.

Ideal or safe medicines are those which after their action in the body is over leave the tissues without causing any harm. An ideal medicine should have four qualities:

- It should be easily available
- It should have the power to eradicate the disease without producing side-effects
- It should be made into the right preparation
- It should possess all proper qualities of taste, energy, and post-digestive effect to produce the desired result

Dosage of Medicines

Right effect depends on correct dosage. Excess doses can cause side-effects, while doses too small will not be effective. Dosage of medicines varies according to constitution, digestive power, strength of the individual, age, disease power, potency of the medicine, and condition of the gastro-intestinal tract.

The Ayurvedic physician Sharangdhara has suggested that for a one month old child the dose should be 125 mg. (one Ratti). This should be increased at the rate of one Ratti per month, up to one year, when the total will be twelve Rattis or about 1.5 gms. The following approximate doses should be used according to different preparations:

Expressed juice of herbs (Swarasa) and herbal wines (Asava or Arishtha) — 20 ml. (½ Pala)

Decoction (Hima, Phanta) — 40 ml. (1 Pala)

Powder (Churna) — 3-5 gms. (½ Karsha)

Medicated Oils, Ghees, and Herbal Jellies (Taila, Ghrita, Avaleha) — 10 gms. (1 karsha)

For Rasayana or rejuvenation therapy a special type of dosage method is suggested. According to this method the dose of the medicine is gradually increased and then gradually decreased in the same manner, as explained in the section on Vardhamana Rasayana.

TIMES TO TAKE MEDICINES (Bhaishajya Kala)

Medicines are taken at different times according to factors like the normal daily variations of the humors, organ reflexes, the state of Agni (the digestive fire), and the stages of digestion. Hence to get the maximum desired effect of the medicine the correct time of administration should be chosen.

ON AN EMPTY STOMACH (Abhakta) — The potency of the drug exerts the strongest action during this time. For strong persons and acute disorders, medicines should be given at this time.

BEFORE MEALS (Pragbhakta) — For treating obesity, Apana Vayu (see glossary) disorders and toning up the intestinal muscles, medicines should be given at this time.

DURING THE MEAL (Madhyabhakta) — For disorders of Samana Vayu (see glossary) this time should be used.

AFTER MEALS (Adhobhakta) — For treating Vyana and Udana (see glossary) disorders, medicines should be given after meals.

This time is also used to treat the diseases above the neck region, which are due to excess Kapha.

MIXED WITH FOOD (Samabhakta) — To suppress the bad taste of medicines, and for children and delicate persons this is the best way to administer them. Similarly this time is used for persons having aversion to medicine, or anorexia, and for treating diseases which have spread all over the body.

BETWEEN LUNCH AND DINNER (Antarabhakta) — This time is suitable to treat the disorders of Vyana Vayu (see glossary).

BOTH BEFORE AND AFTER EATING (Samudga) — For treating diseases like hiccups, trembling, convulsions, and disorders of the lower part of the body, medicines should be given immediately before and after meals.

REPEATEDLY (Muhurmuhu) — For treating diseases like cough, continuous hiccup, dyspnea, vomiting and poisoning, medicines must be given repeatedly.

WITH EACH MORSEL OF FOOD (Sagrasa) — For stimulating digestion and for aphrodisiacs, medicines should be mixed while eating each bite of food.

BETWEEN BITES OF FOOD (Grasantara) — For treating disorders of Prana Vayu (see glossary) this is useful.

AT NIGHT (Nish) — For treating diseases of the head, neck, eye, ear, nose, and throat, medicines should be given at night.

ROUTES OF ADMINISTRATION

Usually medicines are given via the mouth. After digestion and absorption they are circulated by the lymph and blood all over the body. But to achieve specific local action other routes are also used. The general rule is that it is best if we can treat a condition both systemically and locally if possible.

Nose	Medicated nasal drops or powders
Eye	Eye ointments and herbal applications
Ear	For treating diseases of the ear, herbs and oils may be applied at the site
Anus	Enemas
Urethra	Enema is given by this route to treat urinary Infections

Vagina	In vaginal and uterine disorders, as the use of suppositories, swabbing, and douches
Skin	To treat various skin diseases external applications like washes, poultices, plasters, and oils (Lepa, Abhyanga, and Parisheka)

COLLECTION OF HERBS

One should arise before sunrise on an auspicious day. Mondays or Thursdays, the days ruled by the Moon or Jupiter, are particularly good, and when the Moon is waxing. After praying to the sun, a special prayer should be done before the particular herb, plant or tree whose part is to be taken for collection. Then without talking to anyone, the plant or the herb should be collected. The only exception to this is the collection of plants near water, rivers, or lakes. These plants are most potent at night, hence they should be collected at night.

In India, usually all the herbs become potent between the months of October to December, after the rainy season, hence collection should be done during this period. In North America, roots become potent in the fall, leaves and leafy herbs in the spring, and flowers just before they open. In temperate climates individual species may have their special requirements. The exception to this rule is collection of medicines for diarrhea, dysentery, and vomiting. These medicines have a drying nature and should be collected in the month of May–June when the weather in India is hot and dry. The bark or roots of trees should be cut from the north direction.

PHARMACEUTICAL ASPECTS OF AYURVEDA

The knowledge of how to prepare medicines is called pharmaceutics. Correct knowledge of this is an important qualification of an Ayurvedic physician. Basically Ayurvedic medicines are divided into three classes — herbal, mineral, and animal. While considering herbal medicines many factors are taken into account such as which part of the plant is useful — the root, flower, stem, leaves, bark, or exudations like the resin. Similarly the season for collection is taken into consideration. While using mineral substances, the place where they are found, their qualities like color, smell, and form and their varieties are noted. In the case of animal substances the creature's habitat, age, sex, food habits, and the organ or part of the animal used should be properly studied.

We have seen that herbal properties like taste, energy, post-digestive effect, specific action, and various qualities must be taken into account. At the same time action of the medicine on the particular Dosha, organ, or disease condition in the body must also be considered. While preparing any medicine, a physician must know whether the substance is pure or impure. If it is impure the methods of its purification must be known. If a particular substance is not available at a particular season, appropriate substitutes should be known.

PURIFICATION OF MEDICINES

For purification many methods are used such as to cleanse, sort out, peel off, unhusk, polish, strain, filter, distill, or dehydrate the substance. For purification of metals and minerals many processes are used like trituration, boiling in milk or cow's urine, soaking in vinegar, or keeping the substance for a long time in animal products like buttermilk.

The modern pharmaceutical industry requires a range of various chemicals or solvents in its preparation of medicines. The Ayurvedic pharmacy, on the other hand, uses the contact of mineral with heat along with certain purifying herbal substances or juices. The mercurial or gold preparations require many physical and very subtle chemical processes before their final stage is achieved. Ayurveda offers a wide range in pharmaceutical specialties. The most simple procedure consists of crushing the leaves and taking out the juice of an herb. The complex ones require a sequential processing spread over a long period of up to thirty years, like the ancient preparation of Abhrak Bhasma (oxide of mica).

Ayurveda does not use any heavy metals or minerals without such extensive processes to render them humanized or fit for human consumption. In this regard it does use drugs medicinally but in a more careful, complex, and safer manner than modern biomedical usage. Such drugs do not accumulate in the tissues but are discarded once their work is done. In this way Ayurveda can benefit from the great power of minerals without suffering from their side-effects. Ayurvedic medicines thus are much more complex than simple herbal preparations or simple drug preparations. They have an efficacy greater than either and preserve the powers of both.

The most important factor in the preparation of a medicine is Agni or the heat which converts the substance so that it can be accepted by the human body without side-effects and can be easily absorbed. Agni is also important for bringing about the transformation of qualities which are required in various pharmaceutical processes. With the help of heat or Agni, many processes like heating, frying, melting, burning, smoking, cleansing, drying, distillation, digestion, and oxidation can be carried out.

During ancient times, although there was no equipment to measure heat gradations, various grades of heat were specifically described like low, medium, high, very high, and extremely high. For these certain parameters were used like the temperature at which hay burns, at which ammonium chloride melts, or Borax loses its water of crystallization. Also, for controlling temperature at various grades, different heating methods were used like the sand bath, water bath, oil bath, and sulphur-melting bath. They are still in use today. Various qualities of heat were obtained from many different sources like cow dung, sheep dung, horse dung, various types of woods like catechu, coal of different woods, and the husk of rice.

Procedures used — like trituration, moderate contact heating until the powder is liquefied, closed-shell heating, and heating in boiling liquid sulphur — show the portion of the body in which the action of the medicine is likely to take place.

Purification Procedures

In Khalvi preparations various drugs are triturated with liquid extracts of the herbs. An herbal powder is put into a mortar and pestle with the juice of an herb and it is triturated (stirred in a clockwise motion with the pestle) until it is completely dry. This is one Bhavana or procedure. These are done at least seven times. Such medicines act mainly on the upper part of the gastro-intestinal tract, because the heat applied in this process is nothing but friction between mortar and pestle during trituration. The process of trituration is the basis of the other preparations which follow.

In Parpati preparations, first Kajjali or "humanized" Rasa (sulphur and mercury) is prepared. Other herbs and minerals are then added one by one and triturated to create Kajjali powder. The components are next subjected to heat on a hot iron plate, which is just enough to liquefy the combination. Then it is taken out and put on a banana leaf and allowed to cool. As this process requires more heat than the Khalvi group, these medicines do not break down as quickly. They get disintegrated in the middle portion of the gastro-intestinal tract and therefore act on the digestive and absorptive portion of the small intestine. Hence medicines to improve absorption are prepared in this way.

Still further micro-refined products materialize in the process of preparing the Kupipakva group. Kajjali is taken, along with some medi-cines triturated in it, put into a glass shell and fired together usually in sand for twenty-four to seventy-two hours. These are also Rasa or alchem-ical preparations using Kajjali or humanized mercury-sulphur as a base. Here the heat contact is such that the ingredients are put into an almost closed glass shell. The heat applied is much higher than that for the Khalvi group. During this process we get two different products — one at the sublimated portion at the neck of a glass shell or bottle and the other in the sedimented portion at the bottom. Even though both products arise from the same initial ingredients, the substances in the sublimated portion and those in the sedimented portion differ in their elemental constituents. Those found in the neck portion act on the lung, heart, and brain, while those at the bottom are more compact and hence act on pelvic organs like uterus and kidneys.

The Kupi prepared medicines are now refined further, which brings yet a stronger bond between the medicines (sulphur and mercury). In the Pottali group, a sulphur cooking medium is used. The medicines are placed in a cloth bag and immersed into boiling sulphur for up to six hours. Sulphur gives heat from all sides to the particles of the formula suspended in it. These drugs are meant for quicker action, even sublingual, and their action is on deeper tissues often directly through the brain. The best example is Hemagarbha, purified gold.

Preparation of Bhasmas

Oxidation of metals is a specialty of Ayurvedic pharmaceutical processes. The substances resulting are called Bhasmas. These are primarily oxides of the metals but their exact chemical nature is not yet known and may be more than this.

For hard metals (Maharasa) the following procedure is used. Each metallic substance, in the form of a flattened piece, is heated on charcoal and then dipped into oil, buttermilk, cow's urine, kanji (fermented wheat gruel), and a decoction of horse gram. In each of these mediums the metal is heated and dipped seven times. When it is purified the metal becomes very brittle, and another process called Marana is done. The purified metal is put into an earthen shell on to which another earthen shell is made. It is sealed airtight with a cloth dipped in clay. When the shell is dry, it is heated on coals from the wood of special trees or cow dung. Heat is applied for six to eight hours and the Bhasma is thereby prepared. This procedure may be repeated many times for preparing certain Bhasmas.

For such prepared Bhasmas many tests are done to prove that they are ready to be used. These tests are different for different Bhasmas. For example, Copper Bhasma should be put into lime juice and should not turn green. If the Bhasma does not pass the test, it is subjected to repeated firings until it does.

For a lighter mineral (Uparasa) like coral, conch shell, and gypsum, it is heated in the shell for six hours and then it is finished. It requires only one heating.

LIST OF AYURVEDIC PREPARATIONS

Kwatha	Decoction
Phanta	Hot infusion
Hima	Cold infusion
Swarasa	Fresh juice
Kalka	Crushed pulp of the plant
Ghana	Herbal decoction evaporated to solid
Arka	Liquid extracts
Avaleha	Herbal jellies
Asava and Arista	Fermentations or tinctures of herbs
Churna	Powders
Ghrita	Medicated ghee
Kshara	Extraction of alkalis from plants
Lavan	Salts
Guggul	Resins and balsams
Lepa	Pastes
Upanaha	Poultices
Malahara	Ointments
Panak	Crushed fruit and their preparations
Sattva	Active or concentrated herb principles
Taila	Medicated oils
Varti	Suppositories
Guti-vati	Tablets
Bhasma	Herbal oxide ashes
Sara	Resins
Kshira	Exudations
Anjana	Ointments
Dravak	A mixture of various ashes of plants, salts, and alkalies distilled to produce a liquid substance, like Shankhadrava
Druti	Solid substances converted into liquids, like liquefied sulphur

7

THE DISEASE PROCESS
ACCORDING TO AYURVEDA

*The physician who, though knowing the disease, does
not reach the inner self of the patient by the light of his
knowledge, will not be able to treat properly the disease.*

— *Charaka*

CAUSE OF DISEASE

Ayurveda sees the imbalance of the three Doshas of Vata, Pitta, and
Kapha as the immediate cause of all disease. The three Doshas are
damaged or vitiated by disharmonious diet, behavior, and life-style which
result in the imbalance that initiates the pathological changes which
constitute the disease process. In Ayurveda, the etiology of disease has
been described in two broad categories: general factors common to all
diseases, and specific factors behind particular diseases. A third factor
behind disease is recognized in the natural effect of time and the aging
process.

COMMON CAUSES FOR ALL DISEASES
Role of the Senses

One of the most important factors in the disease process in Ayurveda
is the incompatible correlation of the senses with their objects. Sound,
touch, light, taste, and odor are the five sense qualities through which
environmental factors can enter the human body and mind. Excess,
minimal, perverted, and optimal are the possible four types of these
contacts. Out of these only optimal contact is helpful for the maintenance
of health. The three other contacts can cause disease.

It has now been established that the abuse of sound can produce
pathological changes in the blood. Just as sounds or noises that are too
loud can damage the health, the same is true with harmful exposure to, or
abuse of, the other sensory qualities of sight, taste, odor, and touch. Once
the tolerable range is reached everyone should be cautious to avoid
harmful stimuli.

Other medical sciences are also beginning to discover this factor in
diseases. However, it is only in Ayurveda that the role of the senses is

given clear recognition as one of the primary causes of disease. It covers not only physical factors but also psychological factors. It shows the common factors that link physical and mental disorders. If we look at disease only according to external pathogens and do not acknowledge the role of how we use our own senses, we miss much of the real problem. The senses are our real link to the outer world, and our relationship with our environment, healthful or unhealthful, can be measured according to how we use them.

Volitional Transgression

The second main factor in the disease process is volitional transgression or wrong use of the will. In Ayurveda it is known as Prajñaparadha, literally "failure of intelligence." It refers to human weakness by which we resort to substances even after we have experienced them to be harmful. An example is the alcoholic who, even after having experienced a hangover and the side-effects of his drinking, perhaps swearing never to drink again, forgets or ignores this message and starts drinking again. This factor relates to causes from within our psyche that result in defective, excessive, or perverted actions of the body, mind, or speech.

MISUSE OF THE BODY — The misuse of bodily functions occurs mainly through suppression or forced excitation of our natural urges. According to Ayurveda we should not suppress any of our natural bodily urges but should attend to them as they arise. If we suppress them, we derange and weaken the life-force (Prana) and cause our natural impulses towards the healthy function of our bodily processes to be impaired. Nor should we artificially excite these urges through the pursuit of self-indulgence.

MISUSE OF THE MIND — Wrong actions of the mind are due to an increase in agitated (Rajasic) and dull (Tamasic) states of mind, like wrong imagination or lack of attention. This causes the development of fear, grief, anger, greed, infatuation, envy, and other negative emotions which imbalance both the body and mind.

MISUSE OF SPEECH — Misuse with reference to speech refers to indulgence in language that is insinuating, untrue, untimely, quarrelsome, unpleasant, incoherent, harsh, or abrasive. This not only harms others but sets up negative energy patterns within our own body and mind that harm ourselves.

In short, any willful disregard for the natural condition and right usage of things by the mind, followed by wrong action or misconduct is known as volitional transgression. Hence one should use caution not to indulge in overuse or misuse of any function related to mind, body, and speech. Volitional transgression and the wrong use of the senses often go together, as wrong usage of the senses is usually based upon the refusal to acknowledge right usage and natural function.

Effect of Time

The effect of time, or the natural movement of change and transformation, is another cause of disease that no one can avoid. No one can escape the effects of seasonal changes and variations governed by the time factor. Normal as well as abnormal seasonal changes affect the Doshas, mind, and the strength of the body. Similarly every individual has to face the natural process of aging. Disease naturally occurs through the process of growing old. Although to minimize these effects certain methods like seasonal regimens and rejuvenation therapies have been prescribed, one cannot avoid them altogether.

By elaborating these three common causes of disease, Ayurvedic scientists have given clear guidelines for their minimization. The first cause is related to the environment, the second to the psychological complex of inhibition versus indulgence, and the third to the natural fate of every living being.

Factors Responsible for Vitiation of the Doshas

Physical and mental diseases occur due to vitiation of somatic Doshas of Vata, Pitta, and Kapha and due to vitiation of mental Doshas or Rajas and Tamas. Food, drink, or environments with similar properties to the Doshas vitiate them and cause disease. In the same way, behavior of the same nature as the Doshas is also responsible for producing disease.

Ayurvedic texts describe in detail various food items, drinks, and behavior responsible for aggravating Vata, Pitta, and Kapha. Vitiated Doshas, individually or in combination, are capable of producing vitiation in the tissues and give rise to organic or structural diseases. In the same way, specific causes for a wide of variety of diseases are also described in Ayurveda.

CAUSES OF PARTICULAR DISEASES
Specific and Non-Specific factors

The factors producing particular diseases may be either specific or non-specific. One factor may produce several diseases or, on the other hand, several factors may be required to produce one disease. Moreover, in certain cases the cause and the effect may be highly specific, leading to the production of the same disease from the same cause.

Charaka has pointed out the factors responsible for keeping a person free from disease. He states that one who resorts to a wholesome diet and life regimen; who enters into action after proper observation; who is unattached to the pleasures drawn from the satisfaction of the senses; in whom thought, speech, and deeds are happily blended; in whom the mind is controlled and who is possessed of knowledge, austerity, and the love for meditation; such a person seldom gets afflicted with disease.

COMMON PATHOGENESIS OF DISEASES
Branch and Trunk

According to Ayurveda the body is divided into three parts:

THE BRANCHES (Shakha) or four limbs which contain primarily solid tissues

THE TRUNK (Koshtha) containing the gastro-intestinal tract and most of the organs of the body, which has more hollow space than the extremities

HEAD-NECK PORTION which has a structure that can be described as of an intermediate type containing both solid tissues and hollow organs

Formation and Appearance of the Doshas

The food taken by an individual is used up through exercise or work. The food so lost by the body cannot be shown as a weighable or measurable entity. This means that although the food builds the tissues that are measurable, some part of it leaves the body in the form of energy, and that cannot be shown. This energy of movement is the result of previous absorption of food by the body.

Hence Vata Dosha itself is described as the ejectable product of food. Kapha is the ejectable product of nutrient fluids (Rasa) constantly in circulation in the body. Pitta is the ejectable product of hemoglobin blood tissue. Thus it is seen that formation of Kapha and Pitta takes place in solid tissues like plasma and blood, and Vata is measured in terms of the movements of all tissues in the body.

Every day the Doshas appear in the hollow organs of the trunk (Koshtha) from the solid tissues of the branches (Shakha). This occurs according to different factors like the upper, middle, or lower abdominal stages of digestion, of the movement of the Doshas through the cycles of time like day and night, and the process of aging. The appearance of Kapha in the chest and upper abdomen, Pitta in the middle abdomen, and Vata in the lower is also dependent on stimuli, and the quantity available in tissues. But as a physiological process, the Doshas appear in the trunk (Koshtha) and after digestion of food they again go back to the branches (Shakha).

The movement of the Doshas towards the gastro-intestinal tract, their centripetal movement or central pull, is the more natural flow, while the centrifugal force pushing the Doshas towards the solid tissues (Shakha) is observed in pathological states. This means that once the Doshas go toward the branches (Shakha) they do not come back to the gastro-intestinal tract. They remain in the solid tissues and form various diseases.

Excessive exercise, hot atmosphere, too much spicy food, and erratic behavior all push the Doshas toward the branches (Shakha) and cause disease. A person naturally tries to avoid these factors as soon as he notices the hints of an approaching illness. He takes rest, avoids strong stimuli, and keeps himself away from the variety of entertainments that are likely to cause disease.

Physical and mental rest, avoidance of exciting stimuli, and concentration of the mind on recovery aid in the movement of the Doshas back to the gastro-intestinal tract. For this oleation and sudation therapies help. Similarly, control of Vata (Vata Nigraha) through Yoga postures without sudden contraction or relaxation of the muscles is a very important factor in the treatment.

PATHOGENESIS OF SPECIFIC DISEASES

Our bodies are conditioned to adapt within certain limits to variations in the environment and to the stresses to which they are subjected. It is only when the stress exceeds these limits that a disease process begins. Ayurveda divides the disease process into the six stages of disease or the six times for treatment (Shat-Kriyakalas), as these stages determine the nature of the therapies we use to prevent the disease from developing further. These six stages of disease and treatment are:

THE STAGE OF "ACCUMULATION" (Sanchaya) of the Doshas at their sites in the body

THE STAGE OF "PROVOCATION" (Prakopa) of the Doshas when they develop proneness to spread

THE STAGE OF THE ACTUAL "SPREAD" (Prasara) of the Doshas throughout the body

THE STAGE OF "RELOCATION" (Sthana-sanshraya) wherein the interaction of the Doshas with the tissues (Dhatus) takes place along with and their deposition in various parts of the body. In this stage the prodromal symptoms of a disease appear.

THE STAGE OF THEIR "MANIFESTATION" (Vyakti), of the appearance of the characteristic signs and symptoms of the disease

THE STAGE OF "DIFFERENTIATION" (Bheda), of the arising of complications or the occurrence of recovery, terminating cure, disability, or death.

The first three stages — accumulation, provocation, and spread (Sanchaya, Prakopa, and Prasara) — constitute the abnormalities of the Doshas which relate more to systemic and functional derangements than particular diseases. The next three stages — relocation, manifestation, and differentiation (Sthana-sanshraya, Vyakti, and Bheda) — relate to the actual manifestation of the disease and the organic changes occurring in the tissues and various organs of the body. The earlier the physician checks the process of the development of the disease the better. The specific signs and symptoms of the vitiated Doshas in various stages of accumulation, provocation, and spread are clearly described in the texts. The physician is expected to identify the stage a particular Dosha is passing through so that he may be able to prevent further development of the disease process.

In the relocation phase (Sthana-sanshraya) the vitiated Doshas combine with Dushya, the damageable factors or bodily tissues, and vitiate them. This is called "the coming together of the disease causing factors and the sites of disease" (Dosha-Dushya Sammurchhana). The spread of the Doshas to the tissues takes place through the channel systems like the blood vessels, lymph vessels, and cellular spaces.

At some level, in the beginning or during the process of pathogenesis, the Agni or digestive power, metabolism, and assimilation is impaired and a new unwanted product is produced. This toxic accumulation of poor digestion is called "Ama" in Ayurveda. Ama may be produced at any level of digestion, intermediary metabolism, or at the end stages when body tissues are formed. Thus there are five factors of pathogenesis:

- The vitiated Doshas.
- The damaged tissues (Dushya) and the interaction of the Doshas with these sites that they vitiate.
- The movement of the Doshas into the body channels through which nutrient material and waste matter or metabolic by-products normally flow.
- Influence on Agni, the digestive juices, enzymes, and hormones.
- The formation of Ama or impaired and unwanted products of digestion and metabolism.

It is worth noting here that immunity or resistance to disease is considered to be the most important factor for prevention of disease or for reducing the severity of the disease attack. Thus the aim of Ayurveda is to promote health or the natural state of balance, to increase immunity and resistance to disease, and to cure disease.

Knowledge of the pathogenic process is important because it allows us to break or check the spread of the vitiated Doshas from the beginning, from the stage of accumulation, or before the disease manifests itself. When the disease is established such knowledge helps us to cure the disease or gain relief before it becomes chronic and complications start. If the disease is already chronic, its purpose is to limit the disability caused by the disease or to allow for rehabilitation.

STAGES OF DISEASE AND YOGA PROCEDURES

According to Ayurveda, there are five major factors which usually take part in the pathogenesis of every disease. These are:

- Suppression of the digestive fire (Agnimandya)
- The accumulation of Ama or toxins
- Obstruction in channels (Srotorodha)
- Loss of tissue resistance (Dushya-vaigunya)
- Vitiation of the Doshas

Although in the majority of diseases all five factors are involved, there are many diseases which are produced by the predominance of only one of them. A disease like rheumatoid arthritis (Ama-vata) is produced by Ama, while for indigestion it is weakness of the digestive power that plays the predominant role. In ascites, blockage of the channels is the major pathogenic factor. Bronchial asthma is produced mainly by the vitiation of the Doshas. In tuberculosis of the lungs, the loss of tissue resistance is the important factor in formation of the disease. It has been found that along with routine Ayurvedic treatment, if different Yoga procedures are used to remove these pathogenic factors better and quicker results are obtained.

Weak Digestive Fire

Suppression of the digestive fire, defective or low digestive power, plays an important part in many diseases. By increasing the power of Agni or the capacity to convert food properly to tissues, Agnimandya can be completely treated. For this purpose Kapalabhati, Suryabhedana, and

Bhastrika type of Pranayama are very useful. Agnisara process also helps to increase the digestive capacity.

Ama Formation

Formation of Ama takes place because of low digestive power. These toxins occur at two levels — in the gastro-intestinal tract and at the tissue level. To get rid of these toxins Vatasar process is very useful. Patients should be asked to carry out Pranayama with inhalation to exhalation in a one to two proportion.

Blockage of the Channels

Often Ama or excess Kapha gets lodged in channels and causes blockage or obstruction in them. First the patient should be examined properly to ascertain whether Ama is still there or not. After making certain that Ama has been removed, Yogic purificatory actions are performed according to the need. Pavanamuktasana helps to get rid of this obstruction.

Loss of Tissue Resistance

According to different pathologies different organs, tissues, or systems get damaged and lose their tone and power. Different Yogic procedures can be suggested for these. For example, for obesity, Dhanurasana (bow pose) and Halasana (plough pose) are useful. For asthma, Jala Neti and Bhastrika are good.

Aggravated Doshas

According to the dominance of the particular Doshas in a particular disease a group of Asanas are suggested. These have been indicated under Yoga Postures for Different Constitutions.

✳ ✳ ✳

DIAGNOSIS

Ayurveda defines the human being as a combination of the five elements along with the perceiving principle (soul or Atman). The five elements are present in the body in the form of Doshas, tissues, and waste materials comprising the various organs and organ systems. The soul activates the material body. Between these two is the mind along with the five sense organs which coordinates the functions of the soul and the physical body. Thus man has three aspects of his character — physical, mental, and spiritual. The period of time during which all these aspects exist and function together is called life.

These three aspects always try to maintain a perfect coordination and harmony. Such a condition is known as health. But an imbalance in this harmony, even by slight changes in any one of these aspects, makes for ill-health or disease.

It is the duty of the physician to diagnose the disease and to adopt appropriate measures to correct these disorders. A proper diagnosis forms the basis for proper treatment, whereas ignorance of disease or improper diagnosis leads to haphazard or inefficient treatment. There are various methods of patient examination (Rogi-Pariksha).

METHODS OF CLINICAL EXAMINATION

Ayurveda recognizes three means of valid knowledge: authoritative knowledge (Aptopadesha) received from experienced and authoritative individuals, direct perception (Pratyaksha), and inference (Anumana), the conclusions based upon sound reasoning.

Authoritative Knowledge

This is available in three forms: scriptures or knowledge from authoritative texts, oral evidence from recognized teachers or authorities who are learned and speak the truth, and knowledge about the disease available from the patient and his well-wishers.

The mode of obtaining information from the patient is by questioning the patient about relevant conditions. The information so revealed is useful in determining the disease. This examination by interrogation (prashna pariksha) is an essential part of diagnosis and the information should be recorded in writing and analyzed carefully. It can supply information on many important points and should include the patient's name; sex; age; place of residence; occupation; duration of disease; causes of disease; onset; location of disease; nature of disease; symptoms and signs of disease in respect to sound, touch, sight, taste, and smell; aggravation or alleviation of signs and symptoms; after effects; complications and sequela; attempts at treatment; and the effect or result of such remedial measures.

There are many more points that are useful for the physician to know, about which the patient can provide information. The information so given by the patient is called the "patient history" and is recorded in the clinical case sheet in a systematic way under the following headings:

- Chief complaint
- History of present illness
- Past medical history

- Family medical history
- Personal, occupational, and social history

Direct Perception

The knowledge obtained by correlation of the soul (Atman), mind, sense organs, and sense objects is known as direction perception (Pratyaksha). The physician should intelligently apply his senses to examine the patient. The different forms of examination relative to the different senses are as follows:

Examination with the Ear or Auscultation

The intestinal sounds, the sounds of the joints, variations in the voice of the patient or any other sounds occurring in any part of the body, including the cardiac and respiratory sounds, should be examined with the ear or stethoscope.

Examination with the Eye or Inspection

The colors, shapes, proportions and luster, the healthy or diseased look of the body and whatever else can be seen in the body of the patient should be inspected thoroughly with the help of the sense of vision.

Examination with the Sense of Taste

The examination of the patient's body by the sense of taste is prohibited and should be done indirectly by inference, or by various laboratory tests.

Examination by the Nose or by Smell

The smell of the Doshas, tissues, and waste materials in the entire body of the patient should be noted as to whether they are normal or abnormal.

Palpation or Examination by Tactile Sense

The normal or abnormal feelings of the patient's tissues and organs as found in different diseases can be detected with the help of the tactile sense, by hand. Hot and cold, soft and hard, rough and smooth, and other qualities of the tissues and organs may be detected.

Inference

Inference is reasoning on given premises. The state of the digestive fire can be determined by the patient's power of digestion, the patient's strength by the capacity for exercise, the condition of the sense organs by the clarity of perception, the quality of the mind by the power of concentration. The capacity of understanding is revealed by the patients' goals in life, their emotional state by the strength of their attachments, their infatuation by their lack of understanding, their anger by acts of violence, grief by despondency, joy by exhilaration, pleasure from the sense of satisfaction, fear from dejection, vitality by enthusiasm for undertakings, faith by the opinions they hold, intelligence by their power of recollection, character by conduct, and aversion by what they refuse to do. Latent diseases can be revealed by testing with therapeutic or provocative medications. The degree of morbidity of the disease is revealed by the intensity of the provocative factors, the imminence of death by the severity of fatal prognostic signs, the expectation of recovery by wholesome inclinations, and clarity of mind from the absence of disorders.

TENFOLD EXAMINATION OF PATIENT STRENGTH

For adequate management it is essential to evaluate the exact strength of the patient as well as the disease. For this Charaka advocates a tenfold clinical examination (Dashavidha Pariksha).

- Body constitution (Prakriti)
- Pathological condition (Vikriti)
- Tissue vitality (Sara)
- Body build (Samhanana)
- Body measure (Pramana)
- Adaptability (Satmya) to food, herbs, climate, etc.
- Psychic constitution (Sattva)
- Capacity of digestion (Ahara Shakti)
- Capacity of exercise (Vyayama Shakti)
- Age (Vaya)

Body Constitution

The constitution is of seven types as already discussed: Vata, Pitta, Kapha, Vata-pitta, Vata-kapha, Pitta-kapha, and balanced Vata-pitta-kapha. This is because of the relative predominance of the Doshas during fetal development.

Pathological Condition

This is the major object of the clinical examination. Under this heading one has to assess the causative factors, aggravated humors, affected bodily tissues, habitat, time, strength, and signs and symptoms. As the strength of the disease can be assessed only by the consideration of this factor, the entire clinical examination is designed to elucidate its nature.

Tissue Vitality

Broadly speaking, there are seven types of tissues: plasma, blood, muscle, fat, bone, marrow, and reproductive. These are all examined for the assessment of their optimal state along with the examination of the mind. The inference of optimal state of the plasma is examined through the skin. A person having particular tissue vitality does not suffer from diseases affecting that tissue.

Body Build

This refers to the compactness of the tissues like bone, muscle, and blood. Generally it means a well-built body wherein the bones are symmetrical and well distributed, and the joints are well bound with enough flesh and blood. Such persons are strong and those who appear contrary to this are weak.

Body Measurement

Counting the multiples of individual finger (Anguli) units is called Anguli Pramana. From this estimation, the individual's span of healthy life can be assessed. The height of the average healthy individual is eighty-four times their finger-breadth. This factor has already been discussed under Measurement of Body Proportion.

Adaptability

Substances which are homologous or of like nature to the body are known as "Satmya." Those to whom ghee, milk, sesame oil, and all the six tastes are adaptable are strong, tolerant of difficulties, and long lived. Those who have adapted to only a few things and to only one of the tastes are generally weak and short lived.

Mental Nature

The mind is the controller of the body as long as it is in contact with the soul. According to its degree of strength the mind may be graded as either high, medium, or low. Accordingly individuals have three types of psychic constitutions. The psyche is composed of the three Gunas of Sattva, Rajas, and Tamas. Those who are predominant in Sattva possess high psychic strength. Those predominant in Tamas possess low psychic strength. Those predominant in Rajas fall in the middle. The psychic constitution has been described in detail elsewhere.

Capacity for Food

The capacity for food is to be judged from the capacity to ingest and digest food, and by regularity of the appetite.

Capacity for Exercise

The capacity for exercise is judged by the capacity for work. From the capacity for work three degrees of strength — low, moderate, and high — can be determined. Those who have fatigue upon slight exertion are low in strength. Those who do not fatigue even after severe exertion are high in strength. The rest fall in the middle.

Age

During clinical examination the age of the patient has to be confirmed. Age has been broadly divided into three phases: childhood, middle age, and old age. Kapha, Pitta, and Vata energies are more predominant during childhood, middle age, and old age respectively.

EIGHTFOLD PATIENT EXAMINATION

One of the main forms of general patient examination practiced in Ayurveda is the eightfold examination (Ashtavidha Pariksha). The eight factors examined here are pulse, tongue, voice, skin, vision, general appearance, urine, and stool. These provide a good general idea about the nature of the illness and the condition of the patient.

EXAMINATION OF THE PULSE

The term "nadi" literally means a tube or channel through which something flows. Texts dealing with Yoga philosophy use this term for the nerves. In the context of the eightfold examination nadi refers to the arteries. Pulse examination (Nadi Pariksha) is the examination of the arterial pulses at certain points on the body.

The early hours of the morning are the best times for pulse examination. It can be misleading or incorrect if done after the patient has taken food, exercise or bath, after taking intoxicants, having sex, sleep or when afflicted with hunger, thirst, anger, grief, or worry.

The radial pulse at the wrist is the one best suited for examination. The pulse on the right hand is selected for men and on the left hand for women. The physician should place the first three fingers (index, middle, and ring) of his right hand on the pulse at the wrist of the patient. The fingers of the physician should be placed softly but firmly so that even slight movements of the pulse can be felt. The examination is better done three times with an interval of several seconds in between.

The various factors to be noted during pulse examination are pulse rate (Spandana Sankhya), pulse character (Gati) and pulse qualities (Gunas). The pulse rate is described in terms of the number of beats per thirty seconds (pala) or double the amount per minute as follows:

Newborn child	112 per minute
3-7 years	90 per minute
30-50 years	75 per minute

The pulse character is described as resembling the movement of certain animals and birds. Vata pulse is said to be like a snake, Pitta like a frog, and Kapha like a swan.

Pulse qualities like warm, cold, soft, hard, thin, thick, full volume, empty or collapsed, spiral movement etc., can be ascertained by careful palpation.

Abnormal or Disease Pulse

In conditions of Vata aggravation, the pulse resembles the movement of a snake or leech and is irregular, unsteady, and neither hot nor cold. In Pitta conditions, it resembles the movements of a frog, crow, sparrow, crane or quail, and is warm, rapid, thin, and soft. In Kapha conditions, it resembles the movement of a swan, pigeon, dove, cock, peacock, or elephant, and is steady, cold, thick, and full or hard.

EXAMINATION OF THE TONGUE

The tongue provides valuable information on the health or ill-health of a person. It is also important in the diagnosis of digestive disorders. By examining the tongue one can infer the state of Vata, Pitta, and Kapha, the plasma and blood, and the digestive fire. When vitiated by Vata the tongue is dry, rough and cracked. When vitiated by Pitta it is reddish in color with sores or ulcers and a burning sensation. When vitiated by Kapha it becomes coated, white, and slimy. In anemia it loses its normal color and becomes white and smooth. When Agni is impaired it becomes coated with a white layer (Ama) that cannot be removed by washing the tongue.

EXAMINATION OF FECES

The feces gives much information regarding the condition of the Doshas, tissues, and food digested both in healthy and diseased states. Hence Ayurveda advocates its examination as a diagnostic tool generally in all diseases and especially in disorders of the digestive and excretory systems.

If the digestion and absorption of food is normal the stool is [well] formed and floats on water. This indicates that there is no Ama i[n the] system. On the contrary, if digestion is not correct, it does not float o[n] water but is slimy, with various colors and has a bad smell. This indi[cates] Ama in the system. Examination of the feces can also be carried o[ut for] abnormal blood or fat or the presence of parasites.

EXAMINATION OF URINE

Urine is another important waste product of the body and its e[xami-] nation yields much valuable information for the determination o[f] health and ill-health.

The sample of urine should be collected in a clean vessel — p[refera-] bly in a sterilized glass jar, tumbler, or test-tube — directly at the [time of] elimination after avoiding the first few drops.

Sesame Oil Drop Urine Examination (Taila Bindu Parik[sha)

A small quantity of urine is taken in a broad-mouthed glas[s bowl] and kept undisturbed in a place free from wind, sun, and other di[sturbing] factors. A moderate-sized drop of sesame oil is then taken with a stick and allowed to fall on the surface of the urine from a height of two or three inches, gently without disturbing the urine. The condition of the oil drop should be carefully observed for its spread and the different shapes or patterns it assumes. The following interpretations can be drawn from the observations:

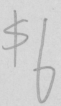

MODE OF SPREAD	PATTERN, SHAPE	CONDITIONS
Floats like a boat	Resembles a snake lengthwise	High Vata
Bubbles appear, splits into small drops	Assumes the shape of an umbrella or ring	High Pitta
Stays like a pearl	Resembles a sieve	High Kapha

EXAMINATION BY TOUCH

This is a method to understand the condition of the various parts of the body in respect to their normal or abnormal qualities. It has not been elaborately dealt with in the texts. It is said that the touch of a person with a Pitta disorder is hot, that of one with a Kapha disorder cold and oily, while that of one suffering from Vata diseases is cold and dry or rough.

EXAMINATION OF THE EYES

Examination of the eyes of the patient also provides much information about the condition of the Doshas. Pitta conditions are revealed by red or inflamed eyes, Kapha conditions by mucus in the eyes or watering of the eyes, while Vata problems manifest by dryness and tremors of the eyes.

GENERAL APPEARANCE

The different systems of the body are examined according to their function and external appearance. For many Ayurvedic doctors this method is more important than pulse diagnosis. Each system, along with the functions and organs relative to it, are examined in various ways, with reference particularly to the predominant Doshas and qualities of damaged or healthy tissues.

EXAMINATION OF DISEASE (ROGA PARIKSHA)

The disease itself must be examined for proper diagnosis. There are five approaches for this:

- Causative factors (Nidana)
- Prodromal symptoms (Purvarupa)
- Signs and symptoms (Rupa)
- Means of alleviation (Upashaya)
- Disease pathogenesis (Samprapti)

Pathogenesis has already been discussed. Upashaya requires some clarification. There are certain diseases where the diagnosis becomes difficult or may not even be possible. In such cases, certain therapeutic tests are done. This is called Upashaya or "means of alleviation." The definition of Upashaya according to Charaka is "the use of medicines, diet, and regimens which are antagonistic directly or indirectly to the causative factor behind the disease, the cause of the disease or both."

In short, the program for the examination of the patient should consist of:

- Factors that aggravate the disease
- Causative factors
- Onset
- Location
- Signs and symptoms
- Pain
- Sound

- Touch
- Color
- Taste
- Odor
- Complications
- Stage of aggravation
- Continuity of disease
- Lessening of disease
- Sequelae
- Name and classification of disease
- Medicines
- Rules of treatment.

The diagnosis of a disease is based on these methods but the teachers have also placed a great emphasis on the three Doshas in practical life. These are useful for both the experienced and beginning practitioner. In this respect Charaka states:

> When classified according to cause, pain, color, site, form, and nomenclature, the number of diseases becomes really countless. A physician need not be ashamed if he is not able to name all diseases, as there can be no definite standardization of nomenclature for all diseases. The same provoked Dosha produces various diseases according to a diversity of causes and its location. Therefore treatment should be initiated after diagnosing the nature of the disease (with the vitiated Dosha and Dushya) and any special causative factors.[1]

The complexity of disease factors, though noted in detail, can be resolved into the patterns of the primary Doshas. In this way Ayurveda can treat diseases in a direct manner that goes right to the cause and does not become concerned with unnecessary details.

8
METHODS OF
AYURVEDIC TREATMENT

He who knows only the theory but is not proficient in practice gets bewildered on being confronted with a patient, just as a coward feels on the battlefield.

Only the wise person who knows both theory and practice is capable of obtaining success, just as only a two-wheeled chariot is useful in the battlefield. – Sushruta

Ayurvedic treatment is defined under the term Chikitsa, which derives from the root "kit," meaning the cure or relief from disease, the removal of its cause. The definition of treatment in Ayurveda is the widest possible for any system of medicine. It is the beneficial usage of medicine, diet, and practices prescribed separately or together. These are described as:

- Contrary to the cause of the disease,
- Contrary to the disease itself, or
- Contrary to both the cause and the disease.
- Similar to the cause of disease,
- Similar to the disease itself, or
- Similar to both the cause and the disease.

This scope covers all the principles of allopathy, homeopathy, and naturopathy. There are forty-two alternate therapeutic approaches arising from the combinations offered by this definition. This explains why Ayurveda does not oppose any of these "pathies" and why it is called "the mother of all medical sciences." Homeopathy, which means literally treatment by similars, and allopathy, meaning literally treatment by contraries, can be regarded, in the words of the founder of Homeopathy, Samuel Hahnemann, "the exact opposite" of each other. But according to Ayurveda both are acceptable alternative approaches. Thus the homeopathic opium that cures constipation and the allopathic opium that causes it both fall within the range of Ayurvedic therapeutic measures.

The Ayurvedic definition of medicine is wide and comprehensive. "Nothing exists in the realm of thought or experience that cannot be used as a medicine (therapeutic agent)." This means that all existing phenomena, physical or psychological, including anger and tranquility, joy and sorrow, fear and confidence, love and hate, food and drink, medicinal substances of mineral, vegetable or animal origin, practices like fasting, massages, postures and exercises, desirable or undesirable experiences or situations, social, climatic or geographical conditions, laudatory or adverse comments, and good, bad or indifferent thoughts have a bearing on health. There is nothing that can be experienced or conceived of which does not influence the body or mind to some degree positively or negatively. Merely hearing the name of a friend or foe can affect the metabolism for better or for worse. Since anything that affects the constitution can be utilized as a therapeutic agent, there is nothing that is not medicine.

Ayurvedic treatment covers a vast field. It not only means relief from disease but bringing the patient back to his normal individual constitution. It includes relief from stress and strain, worry and anxiety. It includes not only medicines but diet, daily routine, atmosphere, and mental health.

The term Kaya-chikitsa is used specifically to refer to Ayurvedic treatment. There are three main words used for the body in Ayurveda: Deha, Sharira, and Kaya. Each carries a specific meaning. Deha derives from the root "dih," which means "that which is nourished." Thus Deha carries the sense of anabolism. The term Sharira is derived from the root "shri," meaning "that which decays." Thus the word Sharira carries the sense of catabolism. The term Kaya is derived from the root "chi" meaning "selection of suitable nutrition," the ability to absorb useful substances and eliminate non-useful ones. This carries the sense of both anabolism and catabolism, i.e. metabolism. The process of metabolism takes place with the help of digestive juices, enzymes, and hormones and so some commentators explain Kaya as Agni or the digestive fire. Thus Kaya-chikitsa means the treatment of the whole body and of Agni, of digestion and metabolism.

PREVENTIVE MEASURES

The preventive aspects of Ayurveda consist of the following three disciplines, which have already been discussed in detail.

First is Personal Hygiene (Swastha Vritta), consisting of the appropriate daily routine, seasonal regimen, and ethical conduct. Swastha means a physically, psychologically, and spiritually harmonious condition. Hence various methods which increase physical, mental, and spiritual strength are included under this branch.

Second is Rasayana and Vajikarana, the use of the rejuvenative and invigorating agents. These are special herbs to prevent aging, strengthen immunity, improve mental faculties, and increase vitality. Vajikaranas are specifically used as aphrodisiacs and fertility improving agents. Such practices require preliminary purification or Pancha Karma treatment.

Third is the practice of Yoga. Though Yoga in itself is a separate discipline, as a form of medicine it is considered part of the rejuvenation (Rasayana) practice of Ayurveda. The regular practice of Yoga keeps both body and mind fit, which provides a feeling of well-being, prevents aging, and inhibits disease.

CURATIVE MEASURES

The curative aspects of the practice of Ayurvedic medicine also consist of three parts: Internal Medicine, External Medicine, and Surgery, which are discussed in detail below. In addition, Ayurveda emphasizes the psychosomatic aspect of medicine as is evident from Charaka's classification of methods of treatment as follows:

- Divine or religious therapy (Daiva vyapashraya)
- Rational or objectively planned therapy (Yukti vyapashraya)
- Psychological or spiritual therapy (Sattvavajaya)

Divine or religious, literally "celestial," therapy is applied to those diseases which are neither purely physical nor psychological and whose causative factors cannot be explained from evident causes. It consists of various subtle, religious, or occult methods to ward off negative influences and to promote those which are good. It includes chanting mantras, the spiritual use of herbs and gems, rituals for giving good fortune (Mangala), offerings of oblations (Bali), offerings in general (Upahara), fasting (Upavasa), pilgrimages (Gamana), performance of prostrations (Pranipata), fire sacrifices (Homa), ceremonial penances (Prayaschitta), and rituals for well-being (Swastyayana). This therapy is not so commonly used today, but it is found not only in Ayurveda but also in the tradition of Vedic astrology (Jyotish) as well as various yogic approaches, particularly teachings of the Tantric order.

Rational or objectively planned therapy means use of scientific medicines along with dietary regimen. It is based upon logic and experience and reflects the Ayurvedic model for understanding the workings of natural forces in body and mind. Most Ayurvedic medical practice today falls within this field and it is most specific to those problems which have a clearly defined physical origin and pathology.

Psychological or spiritual therapy means controlling the mind. It consists of developing the clear or Sattvic quality of the mind for gaining self-knowledge and thereby freedom from desire. It is mainly part of the practice of Yoga but used in Ayurveda to promote longevity, aid in rejuvenation, and for the treatment of disease, particularly for mental disorders.

INTERNAL MEDICINE (Antah-parimarjana)

This is the main discipline in the practice of Ayurvedic medicine. It consists of two primary procedures — Purification (Shodhana) and Palliation (Shamana).

Purification (Shodhana)

Shodhana means radical purification by the elimination of aggravated Doshas (the causative factors for disease) from the body. This is done by the Five Purification practices of Pancha Karma therapy. These methods are explained separately under Pancha Karma and are one of the most significant parts of Ayurvedic treatment.

Palliation (Shamana)

This means gradual reduction of the aggravated Doshas at their respective sites as a means of curing disease or decreasing its symptoms. Disease-causing Doshas when eliminated by Purification therapy (Shodhana) do not recur, but there are chances of recurrence when treated under Palliation therapy. However, it is not always possible to treat diseases with Purification therapy because of various factors. Purification therapy can be very strong and is not always suitable for weak or debilitated individuals. In such cases Palliation is prescribed. Palliation consists of seven factors:

- Kshut — literally "hunger," meaning fasting or light diet
- Trit — literally "thirst," meaning restriction of fluid intake
- Vyayama — exercise of various types
- Atapa-sevana — sunbathing
- Maruta-sevana — taking fresh air and exposure to the wind
- Dipana — taking herbs which increase digestive power

* Ama-pachana — taking herbs which destroy Ama or toxins

These methods lower aggravated Doshas, reduce toxins, and cleanse the channels. They are helpful as a preliminary practice to Purification therapy.

Palliation for Vata

When Vata gets vitiated it is either due to improper nutrition (Dhatukshaya) or obstruction in the channels (Margavarodha). Vata also gets aggravated when Ama is mixed with it and is then called Sama Vata. Palliation therapy can be used for Sama Vata or for Vata aggravation owing to malnutrition. It employs different treatments in each case.

For Sama Vata, the therapy requires herbs to burn up Ama (Ama-pachana) like dry ginger and black pepper, along with herbs to increase the digestive fire (Agni-dipana) like fennel or calamus. Mild exercise is indicated with calming Yoga postures, like most sitting poses. Short term fasting or a light diet is also indicated.

For Vata aggravated by malnutrition, Palliation consists of tonification (Brimhana). Here an adequate nutritious diet consisting of wheat, rice, sweet fruit, root vegetables, dairy products, raw sugar, and nuts is required. For this type of high Vata it is said that "Tonification is as good as Palliation" (see also Tonification in this regard).

Palliation for Pitta

Pitta is aggravated by the increase of hot and sharp qualities in the body. At such times the patient should be massaged with cooling oils like sandalwood prepared in a coconut oil base. Light exercise is good, like swimming in cool water, and a cool and light diet is indicated like ghee, sweet fruit, wheat, mung beans, along with relaxation.

In some conditions, like long-lasting fevers, Pitta brings about an increase of dryness in the body. Here one must remember that this dryness is not the original quality of Pitta but caused by high heat which overcomes the lesser damp quality of Pitta. For such conditions the best Palliation therapy is to give ghee treated with bitter herbs like katuka or barberry.

Palliation for Kapha

For Palliation, Kapha requires strong digestive stimulants like Trikatu, chitrak, turmeric, and dry ginger. Fasting for longer periods of time without food or water is good, followed by a light and dry diet. Strong physical exercise, reduction of sleep, exposure to sun, wind, and heat, and stronger yogic practices including Yoga Kriyas can be carried out.

DIETETICS (Pathyapathya)

Pathya means diet and other regimens which create health and counter disease; Apathya means the contrary, what is not appropriate and aggravates these conditions. Ayurveda lays great emphasis on this principle. It says, "If a man uses Pathya — wholesome diet and life-regimes — there is no need of any medicine; and if the patient indulges in Apathya, or the contrary, the medicines will not work." A large variety of dietetic preparations, largely of a vegetarian nature, are described in Indian medicine relative to different diseases. Ayurveda puts a great emphasis on the caution against incompatible diets and also advocates a tenfold regimen while taking meals. (Note the section on food and diet in this regard)

MODE OF ACTIVITY (Vihara)

Vihara means the practices and routines to be observed during health and disease. For example, in the condition of a fever of recent origin, one should avoid sleeping during the day, baths, oil massage, food, sexual activity, anger and excitement, exposure to the wind, and exercise which can aggravate fevers. One should, on the contrary, take complete rest, keep the mind calm and at ease, fast and so on. In this way Vihara includes various life-style and psychological factors.

SIX MAIN METHODS OF TREATMENT (Shad-upakramas)

Upakrama means methods of treatment. There are three pairs of Ayurvedic therapeutic approaches, six in total: Reduction and Tonification (Langhana and Brimhana), Drying and Oleating (Rukshana and Snehana), and Sudation or Astringent (Swedana and Stambhana). These six methods mark the entire field of therapeutics. The first of each pair — Reduction, Drying, and Sudation methods — are meant primarily for reduction of excess factors in the body, Kapha, and excess body tissues. The second of each pair — Tonification, Oleation, and Astringent methods — increase deficient body tissues, such as are most commonly created by Vata disorders.

For diseases due to lack of nutrition to the bodily tissues like low weight, low energy, and improper growth of the body, Tonification, Oleation, and Astringent methods should be used. For diseases due to excessive nutrition of the body like obesity, atheriosclerosis, hypertension, and Ama conditions, Reduction, Sudation, and Drying types of treatment are used.

REDUCTION (Langhana)

The therapy that produces lightness of the body is called Langhana. This type of therapy is indicated for excess Kapha and Pitta, for diseases caused by Ama and weak digestion, for excess of poor quality tissues like fat, muscle, and bone, and for toxins in the blood. Whenever there is an excess amount of waste products in the body, Reduction therapy is advised. Charaka explains a similar type of therapy under the heading "Asantarpana," described as following the strict dietary restrictions of the Reduction therapy for long periods of time, along with hard work, vigorous exercise, and giving up of comforts.

Reduction therapy has two parts — Palliation (Shamana), and Purification (Shodhana), already described as the two main procedures of Ayurvedic internal medicine. Langhana consists of ten methods, including four types of Purification processes: Vamana (emetics), Virechana (purgation), Asthapana Basti (decoction enemas), and Shiro-virechana (cleansing nasal medications). The remaining six methods of Reduction therapy are Palliation methods: restriction of fluid intake (Trit), exposure to wind or fresh air (Maruta-sevana), sunbathing (Atapa-sevana), taking of herbs to promote digestion (Ama-pachana), fasting, and exercise including Yoga postures.

TONIFICATION (Brimhana)

Tonification therapy is the reverse of Reduction. The line of treatment which increases body weight and strength is called Brimhana. This therapy is indicated for the emaciated, weak or debilitated, and for those in convalescence from chronic illnesses like anemia, sprue, tuberculosis, or other wasting diseases. It is essential for Vata disorders that originate from malnutrition. It is also useful in many Pitta and some Kapha conditions. It is contraindicated in conditions of Ama or toxins, and in febrile diseases.

Tonification therapy consists of a rich diet, tonic herbs, rest and a relaxing life-style. Food prepared with ghee, butter, milk, raw sugar, and jaggery is used. Almonds, pistachios and other nuts are often added. Tonic herbs like shatavari, ashwagandha, bala, and amalaki are taken, particularly the herbal jellies (Prash and Avaleha) prepared from them. The life-style should have no tension or stress, with plenty of rest and enjoyment. For Tonification, herbs indicated under rejuvenation (Rasayana) and invigoration (Vajikaranas) should be taken and mental tranquility should be maintained throughout the course of treatment.

Tonification According To Dosha

VATA individuals require a strong form of tonification. For this, warm sesame oil massage, warm baths, warm clothing, and a warm environment or climate are essential. Nutritive food is essential with dairy products, grains like wheat, nuts, and raw sugars. Tonic herbs like ashwagandha should be taken along with herbs to increase the digestive fire like Trikatu or ginger.

PITTA people require moderate tonification. They should be given massage with cooling oils like coconut. The diet should consist of nourishing food like mung beans, wheat, basmati rice, raw vegetables, and sweet dairy products. Fasting and the use of spices are not good in their case.

KAPHA people require the minimum tonification. As their appetite is not strong, they should eat whole grains like basmati rice, barley, or corn, with a lot of spices like Trikatu, cayenne, or garlic, drink herbal wines (Asava and Arishta) made from ashwagandha, or take tonic herbs like garlic or shilajit.

DRYING METHOD (Rukshana)

Rukshana means the therapy by which the unctuous, sticky, and fatty constituents of the body are dried up or rendered dry. For this purpose food with drying qualities is used. This includes grains like barley and rye, beans like soy and horse gram, and honey that is over six months old. Dry massage with powders of calamus, sandalwood, lodhra, or udumbara is used to remove oiliness from the skin. Decoctions of Dashamula or astringents like catechu can be taken internally.

Drying method is used in those diseases where Kapha is increased due to liquification, as in the common cold, cough with expectoration, and diabetes.

OLEATION (Snehana)

Oleation therapy is the reverse of Drying therapy. The bodily constituents which are dry are rendered oily or unctuous by Snehana. Oleation is carried out with four types of oils: ghee (clarified butter), vegetable oils (like sesame), muscle fat, and bone marrow. Oleation can be administered orally via food and drink, through the rectum by enemas, and through the skin by massage.

This therapy is indicated for Vata diseases due to dryness, and, in rare cases as under Palliation, for Pitta aggravation due to heat and dryness. Oleation therapy is divided into two types — external and internal.

External Oleation

The types of oil massage appropriate for different constitutions has already been outlined under Palliation therapy. Usually Kapha-type people require little oleation. To minimize the heavy quality of Oleation therapy it is better to carry out massage with heating herbs like calamus or camphor that are mixed in a rubbing alcohol base. External oil massage is known in Ayurveda as "Abhyanga," and has been described under daily regimens.

Internal Oleation

This is divided into three types:

- Palliating (Shamana), which is included under Palliation therapy
- Purifying (Shodhana) or oleation done preliminary to Pancha Karma or Purification therapy
- Brimhana or tonifying

For high Vata conditions, tonifying Oleation therapy should be carried out, which is one of the best ways of immediately lowering high Vata. For Pitta and Kapha, medicated oils should be used internally for Palliation. Sesame oil is best for Vata, ghee for Pitta, and mustard oil for Kapha.

SUDATION (Swedana)

Swedana means the procedure to induce sweating or perspiration. It may be brought about by heat or fire (with Agni) or even without application of heat (Niragni Sweda). The types of Swedana where heat is necessary are four; Tapa Sweda (application of dry heat, like heating pads or hot sand), Ushma Sweda (application of steam), Apanaha Sweda (application of hot poultices like wheat flour), and Drava Sweda (use of hot liquids or herbal decoctions externally for baths). These four types are further divided into fourteen types according to the methods and articles used. Heat also may be applied indirectly as via exercise, blankets, sun bathing, or the drinking of herbal wines.

Sudation therapy is applied to all diseases which result from excess cold, oiliness, and those in which poorly-formed tissues are in excess. It is divided into external and internal types.

External Sweating Therapy

This therapy is further divided into either whole-body or partial-body therapies (Sarvanga and Ekanga Sweda). It is used mainly for high Vata and Kapha which are aggravated by cold or damp qualities. For high Pitta this therapy should be generally avoided.

For whole-body sweating therapy for Vata, one should use the medicated steam of anti-Vata herbs like Dashamula, rasna, and nirgundi. For this a special apparatus, or sweat box, is prepared in which the patient can lie or sit comfortably with his head on the outside so it does not get too hot. For Kapha patients, anti-Kapha herbs are used for the steam like lodhra, calamus, or eucalyptus, which are hot and dry in nature. Generally before carrying out external sweating therapy, light oil massage is given. For Kapha, massage with hot, dry herbs like calamus or mustard, again preferably in a rubbing alcohol base, is required.

Partial-body sweating can be done in various ways. For Kapha diseases, dry fomentation with sand can be used, or infrared lamps. For Vata, Nadi Swedana is used. In this the medicated steam of anti-Vata herbs like Dashamula is directed through a hose (nadi), which is used to foment a particular part. This can be done by hooking up a plastic hose to the top of a pressure cooker in which the herbs are cooking.

Internal Sweating Therapy

This is not always as effective as the external method but is easier to use. For this purpose herbs with a hot nature and diaphoretic action are employed, like Trikatu, ginger, cinnamon, or bayberry. Much of the Western and Chinese usage of diaphoretic herbs comes under this type of therapy.

ASTRINGENT METHOD (Stambhana)

The procedure by which the flow of fluids in the body is lessened or checked is called Stambhana, which literally means "stopping." This therapy is indicated in conditions where body fluids like water, blood, urine, feces, sweat, and plasma leave the body in abnormal amounts. Such excess discharges manifest as excess sweating, running of the nose, bleeding, or diarrhea.

For diarrhea, intestinal astringents (Grahi) are used. First hot and pungent types are employed until Ama is digested. For example, first an Ama-burning herb like dry ginger is used and then a more typical astringent like kutaj or alum root. For excess urination (polyuria) as in the case of diabetes, urinary astringents like lodhra are used. For excess bleeding or hemorrhage, hemostatic and styptic herbs are used like turmeric or saffron. In tuberculosis and other wasting diseases of the lungs, plasma (Rasa Dhatu) leaves the body through the phlegm. In such conditions Sitopaladi churna with a large amount of vamsharochana is also good.

The Astringent method is also used for counteracting the side-effects of excess Sudation therapy, which brings on too much sweating. At such times a cold shower or bath, sleeping in the cool air or moonlight, and taking coral or pearl powder is useful.

EXTERNAL MEDICINE (Bahya Parimarjana)

Besides internal medicine there are extensive procedures of external therapy in the form of oleation, sudation, bath, massage, different kinds of medicated gargles, application of pastes, application of powders, and other kinds of therapeutic procedures for the treatment of different kinds of ailments. Such treatments are very popular and as effective today as in ancient times. We have described them under their appropriate places while considering the practices of internal medicine above.

SURGERY (Shastra Pranidhana)

Ayurveda describes a very well planned and systematic surgical discipline which deals with almost all aspects of surgical practice. The texts have described large varieties of sharp and blunt instruments, and splints and bandages for local applications. This has been discussed briefly by Sushrut is under the Eight Branches of Ayurveda.

PSYCHOSOMATIC MEDICINE

Ayurveda is basically a system of medicine with a psychosomatic orientation. The diagnosis and management of each patient is attended by a psychosomatic approach. No treatment is advised without keeping in view the mental nature of the patient, which forms a principal aspect of the clinical conditions. The management of the problem is also advised in view of the psychosomatic factors as is evident by frequent indications of conduct, ethical regime, mantra, and herbs to increase intelligence in the therapeutics.

ASSESSMENT OF TREATMENT

The above-mentioned methods of treatment are employed in consideration of several principles of which the following are important: psychosomatic constitution (Prakriti), age, adaptability (satmya), status of the Doshas, tissues, waste materials, Agnis, channel systems, and Ojas of the patient. The specific medicines, their dosages and modes of administration are to be suitably selected in each individual case depending upon such factors. The degree of success of treatment can be measured by the following indications:

- Relief from the pain of the disease
- Improvement of voice and complexion
- Normalization of body weight
- Increase in strength and vitality
- Desire for food and improved appetite
- Relish while eating
- Timely and proper digestion
- Sleep at the proper time
- Absence of fearful dreams or disturbed sleep
- Feeling of happiness and vitality upon awakening
- Proper elimination of urine, stool, and flatus
- Lack of impairment of mind and senses

9
PANCHA
KARMA

This five-fold Purification therapy is a special form of treatment in Ayurveda. These procedures which permanently eliminate the excessive Doshas or biological humors from the body consist of the following:

1. Vamana, herb induced emesis
2. Virechana, herb induced purgation
3. Asthapana Basti, medicated decoction enema
4. Anuvasana Basti, medicated oil enema
5. Nasya, nasal intake of medication

According to Sushruta, Rakta-moksha or therapeutic blood-letting is also included.

ACTION OF PANCHA KARMA

Day and night and during the digestive process, the Doshas move into the gastro-intestinal tract (Koshtha) from the tissues (Shakha). The body naturally tries to throw away unwanted substances through these gastro-intestinal secretions. Certain portions of the digestive tract are the main sites of secretion for the Doshas: the stomach for Kapha, the small intestine for Pitta, and the large intestine for Vata. This natural process of the appearance of the humors in certain parts of the gastro-intestinal tract is enhanced by Pancha Karma. Thus excess humors are removed from the body.

As the humors and tissues (Doshas and Dhatus) are related to each other, these discharge procedures affect the tissues indirectly by the strong elimination of the related humors. For example, the pronounced elimination of Kapha by herb-induced emesis causes an effect on the nutrient tissue-fluid pool, containing water and electrolytes, plasma, muscles, and fat. The large elimination of Pitta by selective purgation similarly causes an indirect effect on the total coloring material in the body. Basti, medicated enema, is a somewhat different manner, as it is meant to nullify excess Vata. Basti contains warm oleating substances. During its long contact with the membrane of the large intestine it separates the sticky layers of solid fecal matter and by thus enhancing better absorption ultimately nourishes all the tissues. Nasal medications (Nasya) clean the sinuses and thereby improve the function of the sense organs.

Thus this entire group of purification procedures is based upon promoting the body's natural methods of eliminating unwanted substances. These techniques are designed to take advantage of temporary phases of greater secretion or absorption at the related mucous membrane sites. If these procedures are carried out without certain preparatory practices, the body tissues are adversely affected.

OBJECTIVE OF PANCHA KARMA

This therapy can be used to achieve the following three objectives.

Health Maintenance

As part of regular seasonal regimens this therapy is advised for all individuals, even the most healthy. Due to seasonal changes the Doshas get vitiated. These vitiated Doshas can cause disease if they are not removed at the proper time. Hence in the rainy season Basti or medicated enema is advised to alleviate the normal aggravation of Vata. In the winter season, Vamana or Emesis is prescribed to remove excess Kapha. In the summer season, purgation is given to remove excess Pitta.

Adopting these regimens to a four season climate, Vata should be eliminated in the late fall, Kapha in the early spring, and Pitta in the summer.

Treatment of Disease

This procedure should be carried out according to the excess Doshas prevalent in the particular disease. In acute diseases, if the Doshas are removed at the proper time the disease attack can be immediately arrested. In chronic diseases various toxins stick to the organs and cells. Unless these toxins and excess Doshas are first removed by Pancha Karma, the treatment cannot benefit the patient.

Preparation for Rejuvenation or Virilization Therapies

Both these therapies are nothing but selective tissue-enriching programs. To achieve the best results, the body must be purified first by Pancha Karma procedures.

PREPARATORY PRACTICES

For Pancha Karma these are Oleation and Sudation (Snehana and Swedana). With these two procedures the Doshas localized in the tissues and skin (Shakha) are brought to the gastro-intestinal tract (Koshtha) where they can be easily eliminated. The advantage of Oleation therapy is that it makes the main procedures of Pancha Karma less exhausting to the patient. Similarly the gastro-intestinal tract, which has to produce more secretions, gets protection first. During Sudation therapy the channels, openings, and pores of the body are widened so that the secretions (Doshas) can be brought through them easily into the gastro-intestinal tract for elimination. Sudation helps liquefy the Doshas so that their centripetal propulsion is carried out with minimum resistance.

In short, Oleation is for protection of the retainable tissues. It loosens the Doshas which are sticking to the walls of minute channels and creates a centripetal force, while Sudation helps mainly for liquefaction and opens the channels as well as pores for the movement of the Doshas toward the gastrointestinal tract.

Oleation

For this practice, substances like ghee (clarified butter) or sesame oil are used. These substances are chosen according to constitution, disease, and predominance of Doshas. For Vata conditions sesame oil is usually chosen, and for Pitta and Kapha ghee is used. Light diet or fasting is also recommended. Oleation is done on a daily schedule of gradually increasing dosage, until the signs of optimum oleation appear on the body. These are as follows:

- Oily appearance of skin (without any oil being externally applied)
- No white marks appearing after scratching the skin
- Disgust for oleating substances
- Appearance of oil in the stool, along with softness of the stool
- Appearance of lightness in the body

The initial oral dose for Oleation be about 25 gms. as a single dose or the quantity that can be digested within six hours. This is the minimum dose. The medium dose is 37.5 gms. or the quantity which can be digested within twelve hours, and 50 gms. or the quantity which can be digested within twenty-four hours is regarded as the maximum dose. According to original dryness or oiliness of the digestive tract, the period required to achieve optimum oleation varies from three to seven days.

Sudation

This is a therapy by which a person is made to sweat. Generally it is done after Oleation. It has four types:

- By direct application of heat — with electrical fomentation pads, or by heated cloth, sand, wheat flour, or salt in bandage form.
- By applying medicated poultices. This method is comparable to antiphlogistic treatment.
- By steam — like in a steam bath. The only difference is that steam should be prepared from medicated herbs.
- By having the patient take a bath in which hot decoctions of various herbs are mixed with the water.

After Sudation is completed, the patient should be given a light massage and bath and then take a short rest.

PRIMARY PRACTICES
1. EMESIS, VAMANA

This is the therapy of choice for the elimination of excess Kapha from the body through the mouth. The herb of choice is Randia dumetorum seeds, also called emetic nut. Commonly a mixture of this herb with calamus and licorice is used.

Indications and Contraindications

Vamana is indicated in Kapha predominant diseases like cough, asthma, repeated colds, dyspnea, diabetes, nausea, loss of appetite, indigestion, and certain mental diseases like epilepsy.

It is contraindicated for children, the elderly, debilitated, very weak patients, and in certain conditions such as stomach ulcers, trauma to the lungs, heart disease, and abdominal tumors.

Procedure

First the patient is given a course of Oleation and Sudation. Then, prior to the main treatment day, he is given Kapha-aggravating food (Abhishyandi) like rice with yogurt. Due to the preparatory treatment, the vitiated Doshas situated in the distant channels have been loosened and their centripetal activity starts.

Then the patient is asked to sit on a low stool, and his body is covered with a clean towel. He is asked to drink 1 to 3 liters of a warm decoction of licorice. The bulk of the stomach contents is increased by this secretion-promoting herb. Then he is given the main medicine to provoke vomiting. For this calamus powder, licorice, and the powder of the seeds of Randia dumetorum — each 1 gm. — is taken with honey. This is a strong secretion-promoting mixture, hence the Doshas are further stimulated to enter the gastro-intestinal tract. This is indicated by the sign of perspiration on the forehead. Vomiting starts shortly thereafter, and thus the vitiated Doshas — mainly Kapha and Pitta — are eliminated from the body.

When the patient feels the sensation of nausea, he is instructed to vomit without undue strain. The head should be supported while the patient is actually vomiting. First the patient will vomit white, sticky, and slimy substances and then yellow bile comes out. At this stage vomiting usually stops automatically. The amount vomited is evaluated as to whether it is maximum, medium, or minimum. These are judged from the number of vomitings and the total quantity of vomit expelled during the therapy.

Number of Vomitings	Quantity Expelled
4 Minimum	325 cc.
6 Moderate	650 cc.
8 Maximum	1,300 cc.

However, the symptoms of proper elimination are more important than the quantity expelled or the number of vomitings. These are a feeling of lightness in the body, increased digestive power, decrease in the symptoms of the disease for which the emesis was prescribed, and the automatic stopping of vomiting after the expulsion of the Doshas.

After treatment the patient should clean up and be allowed to rest. Then he may be asked to smoke a mixture of medicated herbs and resins for removing residual Kapha in the upper respiratory tract. When he feels hungry he should take a bath. Then starting with kicharee or basmati rice, he should very slowly be given a diet of increasingly heavier quality, in such a way that on the seventh day he can return to his normal diet.

2. PURGATION (Virechana)

With selective purgation, vitiated Pitta and Kapha are eliminated from the body. For this procedure also the patient is first given Oleation and Sudation therapies. Purgation can be done three days after emesis, but it can also be given directly if emesis is not required.

Indications and Contraindications

Purgation is indicated in skin diseases, chronic fevers, enlargement of the liver and spleen, jaundice, erysipelas, glandular swelling due to vitiated blood, and various diseases of toxic blood due to Pitta, like stomatitis, glossitis, and hyperacidity.

It is contraindicated in children, very old and weak patients, when there has been bleeding through the rectum, ulcers of the large intestine, fissure in the anal canal, diarrhea or dysentery.

Procedure

The medicine of choice in this therapy is a decoction of Draksha, aragwadha, and haritaki, 12 gms. each, and katuka, 6 gms. First make a decoction of these herbs in water and then take two ounces of this decoction and mix it with two ounces of castor oil. This is an ideal medicine for purgation. Among Western herbs, rhubarb root is particularly useful. It can be taken as a powder in dosages of 5–10 gms. along with a quarter that amount of cardamom.

Purgation should be carried out from four to six hours after sunrise. The patient is asked to drink the medicine prepared for purgation. Soon purgation starts due to its secretion-promoting action. Three degrees of elimination by purgation have been described as follows:

Motions	Expelled Quantity
5 Minimum	500 cc.
8 Moderate	1,000 cc.
10 Maximum	1,600 cc.

Feeling of cleanliness in the channels and sense organs, lightness in the body, and increase in appetite (after some time) are the indications of proper elimination by purgation. During the procedure, the patient first passes liquid fecal matter and urine, then mucus, and then yellowish colored Pitta (bile).

After treatment the patient should rest. Then, as in Vamana therapy, light food should be taken. This consists of starting with a light diet like vegetable soup and then slowly increasing the diet to a heavier quality, so that on the seventh day the patient can return to his normal diet. On the ninth day, Basti treatment can be started.

3.–4. MEDICATED ENEMAS, BASTI

In this procedure medicated oils and decoctions are introduced into the large intestine with the help of an enema bag. The word Basti means the urinary bladder. In ancient times the urinary bladders of various dead animals were used for this purpose.

The Four Ways of Classifying Enemas

1. According to the site where they are applied:
   * Rectum
   * Vagina
   * Urethra
   * A wound cavity

2. According to the substance used:
   * Cleansing (Niruha)
   * Oleating (Anuvasana)
     In Niruha Basti, salt, honey, oils, pastes, and decoctions of herbs are used. This is also known as Asthapana Basti. According to the variation of substances used, this Basti is further classified into Yapana, Brimhana, etc. In Anuvasana Basti, only sesame oil or medicated sesame oil is used.

3. According to therapeutic action:
   * Shodhana — for Purification
   * Lekhana — for reducing excess tissues
   * Snehana — for Oleation
   * Brimhana — for increasing deficient tissues in the body
   * Shamana — for Palliation
   * Doshahara — to remove particular Doshas

4. According to the course of treatment:
   * Karma — total course of thirty Bastis. In this course first one Anuvasana Basti is given, then alternately twelve Niruha and twelve Anuvasana are given, and finally five Anuvasana are given.
   * Kala — total course is sixteen Bastis. First one Anuvasana, then alternately six Niruha and six Anuvasana are given, and finally three Anuvasana.
   * Yoga — total course of eight Bastis. First one Anuvasana, then alternately three Anuvasana and three Niruha, and finally one Anuvasana are given.

Indications and Contraindications for Cleansing (Niruha) Enema

This is indicated in diseases of Vata especially when it is vitiated due to obstruction in the channels; e.g. conditions like pain in the abdomen, chest, pelvic region, eye, ear or legs, headache, cardiac pain, hemiplegia, facial paralysis. Usually Dashamula (the ten roots) decoction is used.

It is contraindicated in conditions of indigestion, obstruction or perforation in the intestines, for very old or debilitated patients, for toxins (Ama) in the gastro-intestinal tract, diarrhea, and vomiting.

Indications and Contraindications for Oily (Anuvasana) Enema

The indications are largely the same as those for Niruha Basti. It can also be used for diseases of Vata due to tissue loss (wasting and debilitating diseases).

Its contraindications are hemorrhoids, excessive Kapha in the gastro-intestinal tract, low digestive power, and ascites.

Preparation of Cleansing Enema

To prepare the mixture for this type of enema, one must follow strictly a sequence of mixing various ingredients. First add honey and rock salt, and mix properly. Then add to this the proper oleating material, sesame oil or ghee, again mixing properly. Then add to it a fine paste (Kalka) of herbs, and finally add to it the medicated decoction. The whole mixture, when thoroughly mixed, should be heated to body temperature over water vapor. Then pour these contents into an enema bag. The quantity of the total mixture may range from 700 to 1200 cc. depending upon the age, disease, and condition of the patient.

Procedure for Cleansing Enema

This procedure should be carried out four to six hours after food has been taken and preferably early in the morning or the evening. The patient should lie on a bed with the head low and in the left-lateral position. He should be asked to extend his left leg, with the right leg taken near the abdomen by folding it. He should keep his left hand below the head. Then a small amount of oil should be applied to the rectum as well as to the nozzle of the Basti applicator. After this the nozzle should be inserted slowly into the rectum and the balloon should be squeezed. When all the contents of the Basti have entered into the large intestine, the nozzle should be slowly withdrawn. The medicated contents should be retained in the intestine for some time and then allowed to come out again along with the fecal matter, and excess Pitta and Kapha. The patient should be asked to use a bedpan.

After treatment the patient should be given rest. Then he is given warm water and when hungry should be given a diet consisting of grains, milk, and other rich substances.

Preparation of Oil Enema

For this medicated or plain sesame oil is used. The main procedure and post-enema treatment is the same as that of Niruha Basti. The only difference is that here the quantity being small, from 60 to 100 cc., a large plastic syringe can be used. The contents of the enema, being small in quantity, do not cause any harm to the patient even when retained in the intestine for more than twenty-four hours.

5. NASAL MEDICATION, NASYA

In this procedure medicated oil or powder is administered into the nose. In this way the vitiated Doshas above the region of clavicle — in the head and neck — are eliminated through the nose. Hence this therapy is specifically advised for head and neck diseases.

Types of Nasya

There are three ways of differentiating the various forms of nasal medications.

1. According to action:
   - Purification (Shodhana) or Purgation (Virechana) — for the elimination of Doshas
   - Palliation (Shamana) — for the reduction of Doshas
   - Tonifying (Brimhana) — for subsidence of Vata

2. According to the substance used:
   - Avapida — medicines put into the nose like herbal extracts
   - Navana — instilling liquids into the nose like milk and oils
   - Dhuma — inhaling the smoke of various herbs
   - Virechana-Dhumapana — employing medicinal powders into the nose with a special apparatus

3. According to the dose:
   - Pratimarsha — a dose of only 2 drops in each nostril
   - Marsha — 8 to 32 drops in each nostril.

Indications for Liquid Nasya (Avapida and Navana)

This is a Palliation type of Nasya indicated in all Vata-caused diseases of the head, ear, eyes, and nose. It is also useful in Vata and Pitta-caused diseases of the mouth, falling of hair, or dryness of the throat; usually Anu Taila is used for this purpose.

Indications for Dhuma and Dhumapana Nasya

Dhumapana Nasya is a purificatory type of Nasya indicated in all diseases where Kapha is to be eliminated from the head region, as in sinusitis, heaviness in the head, epilepsy, or loss of voice. For this purpose, the powder of rock salt, garlic, dry ginger, calamus, and black pepper is used. For Purification type of smoking therapy (Dhuma Nasya), guggul and other medicated resins are used.

Procedure for Nasya

After attending to the daily morning routine, the patient is asked to clean his teeth and mouth, then he is asked to smoke the medicated herbs. Later on, Pañchaguna or Bala oil is applied to his forehead and face. Then he is given fomentation by Tapa Sweda method on these parts. Lastly, light massage is performed on the frontal part of the head, throat, and cheeks.

Nasya of the liquid type can be carried out when the patient is sitting or lying on the bed. If the patient is lying in bed, then the head-end of the bed or table should be lowered a little. The patient should be asked to extend his neck so that his nostrils face upwards. Then medicated oil should be placed into the nostrils. Soon secretions begin to come from the nose. Afterwards there is a sensation of lightness in the head and the disease symptoms are reduced. Nasya, if properly done, improves the functions of all the sense organs.

After treatment, mild fomentation and massage should be applied over the forehead, cheeks, and throat. The patient should clear the throat of any residual amounts of the Nasya medication, and should gargle with hot water and inhale medicated smoke.

THERAPEUTIC BLOODLETTING (Raktamoksha)

Sushruta includes both types of Bastis in one category and considers bloodletting as the fifth purificatory procedure of Pancha Karma. Sushruta gave much importance to the blood, perhaps because he was a surgeon. He considered blood to be a fourth Dosha in the body. Pure blood has life-giving value, while impure blood can create or spread diseases. Hence impure blood should be removed from the body. Sushruta has emphasized this therapy as Charaka has given importance to Basti.

Pitta Dosha has an affinity with the blood. Hence when it is vitiated and cannot be treated by the usual medicines, bloodletting can be helpful. Hence it is the therapy for diseases due to both vitiated blood and Pitta.

Bloodletting is indicated for diseases not amenable to hot and oily therapeutic measures (as most Vata diseases), to hot and dry therapies (as most Kapha diseases), or to cold and dry measures (as most Pitta diseases). It is indicated for diseases due to simultaneous vitiation of blood and Pitta (Rakta-Pitta).

Types of Therapeutic Bloodletting

1. With sharp instruments:
   - Prachhana — taking quick sharp incisions
   - Siravyadha — venesection

2. With blunt instruments (like the application of leeches)

Usually when blood and Pitta caused diseases are widespread, venesection is used, and when the disease is localized, leeches are used. Conditions treated by bloodletting include skin diseases like erysipelas, scabies, eczema, pimples, abscesses, and vitiligo; inflammatory diseases like stomatitis, gingivitis, and hemorrhoids; and liver diseases like jaundice and ascites.

This procedure is to be carried out in October or just before the winter season. Venesection is performed with a simple syringe with a No. 18 needle or with the help of a bloodletting apparatus. 300 cc. of blood are taken from an adult patient. The patient should first be prepared with proper Oleation and Sudation.

When leeches are used, the particular part of the body where leeches are to be applied should be thoroughly washed with water (disinfectant drugs should not be applied to the skin). Then a scratch should be made or a drop of milk should be put on the skin where a leech is to be applied. As soon as the leech starts sucking the blood, it should be covered with a damp gauze. After sucking sufficient blood, the leech automatically separates from the skin. The small wound made by the leech should be dressed with medicated oil and then firmly bandaged.

10
MARMA POINTS:
AYURVEDIC PRESSURE POINTS

Marma points are important pressure points on the body, much like the acupuncture points of Traditional Chinese Medicine. One finds the first reference to them in the *Atharva Veda,* and they are elaborately dealt with by Sushruta. Knowledge of these sensitive anatomical points was applied in war for harming the enemy or protecting oneself. This knowledge became an essential part of training for surgeons, as injury to these points can produce death or disability.

A Marma point is defined as an anatomical site where flesh, veins, arteries, tendons, bones, and joints meet together. As the technique of massage developed, these points were used for stimulating internal organs and systems of the body. Marma points are classified according to the different areas on the body where they occur, the tissue of which they are composed, and the effects which are felt if they are injured.

Like the Chinese acupuncture points, Marma points are measured by the finger units (Anguli) relative to each individual. Their size is measured by finger inches, and their location determined by them. However the Marma points differ from acupuncture points in that a number of Marmas are larger in size and mark areas from one to eight finger units in diameter. Thus indicating an area, rather than a point, their definition is often more general.

NUMBER OF MARMA POINTS
By Region

22	Upper limbs	22	Lower limbs
12	Abdomen and Thorax	14	Back and Trunk
37	Head and Neck		

By Structure

11	Muscular	41	Blood vessels
27	Ligaments	20	Joints
8	Bone		

By Signs (if injured)

9	Causing instant death (Sadyaha Pranahara)	8	Painful (Rujakara)
33	Causing death in time (Kalantara Pranahara)	44	Causing Disability (Vikalatvakara)
3	Causing death if hit by a foreign body like a bullet (Vishalyaghnakara)		

EXPLANATION OF SANSKRIT MARMA NAMES

Most of the Marmas are named after their location or function. Hence their names help identify them. Many of these points can be treated either at the front or the back of the body part which relates to them.

HANDS AND LEGS

Talahridaya	Heart or center of the palm of the hand or sole of the foot
Kshipra	Quick, owing to its immediate effects
Kurccha	A knot or bundle of muscles or tendons at the base of the thumb or big toe
Kurcchashira	The head of kurccha, at the base of the hand or the foot
Manibanda	Bracelet, as it goes around wrist
Gulpha	Ankle joint
Indrabasti	"Indra's bladder," mid-forearm and mid-calf
Kurpara	Elbow joint
Janu	Knee joint
Ani	The lower region of the upper arm or leg
Urvi	"The wide," the wide mid-region of the thigh or forearm
Lohitaksha	"Red eyed," the lower frontal insert of the shoulder joint and leg joint
Kakshadhara	"What upholds the flanks," the top of the shoulder joint
Vitapa	The perineum, where the legs are connected to the trunk

ABDOMEN

Guda	Anus
Basti	Bladder
Nabhi	Navel

THORAX

Hridaya	Heart
Stanamula	Root of the breast
Stanarohita	Incline (or upper region) of the breast
Apastambha	A point on the upper side of the chest said to carry the Prana or life-force
Apalapa	"Unguarded," the armpit or axilla

BACK

Katikataruna	"What arises from the sacrum," the center of the buttocks
Kukundara	Marking the loins, on either side of the posterior superior iliac spine
Nitamba	The upper region of the buttocks
Parshwasandhi	The joint of the sides, the side of the waist
Brihati	"The large" or broad region of the back
Amshaphalaka	The shoulderblade
Amsa	The shoulder

NECK

Manya	"Honor," perhaps owing to its connection with the voice
Nila	"Dark blue," from the color of the veins at this point
Sira Matrika	"The mother of the blood vessels," from the arteries to the head that flow through this region
Krikatika	The joint of the neck

HEAD

Vidhura	"Distress," from its sensitive nature
Phana	"A serpent's hood," the side of the nostrils
Apanga	The outer corner of the eye
Avarta	"Calamity," from its sensitive nature
Shankha	"Conch," the temple
Utkshepa	"What is thrown upwards," as it is above the temple
Sthapani	"What gives support"
Shringatakani	"Places where four roads meet," the soft palate of the mouth
Simanta	"The summit," the skull and surrounding joints
Adhipati	"The overlord"

TABLE OF MARMA POINTS

NAME (Extent in Finger Units)	No.	Site	Location	Composition	Effects of Severe Injury	Importance in Treatment
HANDS AND LEGS						
TALAHRIDAYA ½ Anguli	4	In Center of Palm & Sole	On both Palms & Soles	Muscular	Slow Death	Stimulation of Lung
KSHIPRA 4 Anguli	4	On both Hands & Feet	Between Thumb & Index Finger, and First & Second Toes	Tendon	Slow Death	Stimulation of Lung
KURCCHA 1 Anguli	4	Both Palms & Soles	2 Anguli above Kshipra Marma, root of Thumb	Tendon	Disability, Pain, Tremors	Kurccha Marma on Sole controls Alochaka Pitta (eyes)
KURCCHASHRA 1 Anguli	4	Both Palms & Feet	1. Just below Wrist Joint 2. At center of the Heel below Gulpha Marma	Tendon	Pain	
MANIBANDA 2 Anguli	2	Both Hands	On Wrist Joint	Joint	Pain	
GULPHA 2 Anguli	2	Both Hands	On Ankle Joint	Joint	Pain	

NAME (Extent in Finger Units)	No.	Site	Location	Composition	Effects of Severe Injury	Importance in Treatment
INDRABASTI ½ Anguli	4	Both Mid-forearm & Mid-calf regions	In the center of area	Muscular	Anemia, slow death	Stimulation of Agni (digestive fire) and small intestine
KURPARA 3 Anguli	2	Both Hands	On the Elbow joint	Joint	Disability	Stimulation of Liver and Spleen
JANU 3 Anguli	2	On both Legs	On the Knee joint	Joint	Disability	Stimulation of Liver and Spleen
ANI ½ Anguli	4	On Arms & Thigh	3 Anguli above Kurpara and Janu	Tendon	Disability and swelling on the Thigh	
URVI 1 Anguli	4	Upper Arm& Thigh	In the middle of upper Arm or Thigh	Blood vessel	Disability, atrophy of Thigh muscles, anemia	Stimulaltion of Udakavaha Srotas
LOHITAKSHA ½ Anguli	4	Armpit & Inguinal region	Joint of groin or shoulders	Blood vessel	Disability, paralysis due to blood loss	

NAME (Extent in Finger Units)	No.	Site	Location	Composition	Effects of Severe Injury	Importance in Treatment
KAKSHADHARA 1 Anguli	2	Front Arm	2 Anguli above Lohitaksha	Ligament of Shoulder joint	Disability	
VITAPA 1 Anguli	2	Front of the Abdomen	2 Anguli below Lohitaksha, at the root of the Scrotum	Inguinal	Disability, impotence	
ABDOMEN						
GUDA 4 Anguli	1	Around Anus	Around Anus	Muscular	Sudden death	Stimulation of First chakra, Reproductive, Urinary & Menstrual systems
BASTI 4 Anguli	1	Abdomen	In between Pubic Symphysis & Umbilicus	Ligament	Sudden death	Control of Kapha

NAME (Extent in Finger Units)	No.	Site	Location	Composition	Effects of Severe Injury	Importance in Treatment
NABHI 4 Anguli	1	Abdomen	Around Umbilicus	Ligament	Sudden death	Control of Small Intestine & Pachaka Pitta
THORAX						
HRIDAYA 4 Anguli	1	Chest	Middle of Sternum	Blood Vessel	Sudden death	Control of Sadhaka Pitta, Vyana Vayu
STANAMULA 2 Anguli	2	Chest	Below the Nipple	Blood Vessel	Slow death	
STANAROHITA $\frac{1}{2}$ Anguli	2	Chest	2 Anguli above Stanamula	Muscular	Slow death	
APASTAMBHA $\frac{1}{2}$ Anguli	2	Chest	In midline between Nipple & Collar bone	Blood Vessel	Slow death	
APALAPA $\frac{1}{2}$ Anguli	2	Chest	Lateral side of Stanarohita	Blood Vessel	Slow death	

NAME (Extent in Finger Units)	No.	Site	Location	Composition	Effects of Severe Injury	Importance in Treatment
BACK						
KATIKATARUNA ½ Anguli	2	On Buttocks	Center of Hip	Bone	Slow death	Control of Adipose tissue
KUKUNDARA ½ Anguli	2	Back	On each posterior superior Iliac spine	Joint	Disability	Control of Second chakra
NITAMBA ½ Anguli	2	Back	4 Anguli above & lateral to Kukundara	Bone	Slow death	
PARSHWASANDHI ½ Anguli		Back	2 Anguli above Nitamba	Blood vessel	Slow death	
BRIHATI ½ Anguli	2	Back	2 Anguli below lateral side of spine	Blood vessel	Slow death	Control of third chakra
AMSAPHALAKA ½ Anguli	2	Back	On Scapula bone above Brihati	Bone	Disability, atrophy of Shoulder muscles	Control of fourth chakra

NAME (Extent in Finger Units)	No.	Site	Location	Composition	Effects of Severe Injury	Importance in Treatment
AMSA ½ Anguli	2	Back	4 Anguli above Amsaphalaka, between Shoulder and Neck	Ligament	Disability, frozen Shoulder	Control of fifth chakra
NECK						
MANYA 4 Anguli	2	Neck	Posterior side of Larynx	Blood vessel	Disability	Control of Blood
NILA 4 Anguli	2	Neck	Anterior side of Larynx	Blood vessel	Disability	
SIRA MATRIKA 4 Anguli	8	Neck	Four Arteries on each side of Neck	Blood vessel	Sudden death	
KRIKATIKA ½ Anguli	2	Neck	Junction of Head and Neck	Joint	Disability	

NAME (Extent in Finger Units)	No.	Site	Location	Composition	Effects of Severe Injury	Importance in Treatment
HEAD						
VIDHURA 1/2 Anguli	2	Neck	Below both Ears	Tendon	Disability, Deafness	
PHANA 1/2 Anguli	2	Face	On both sides of Nostrils	Blood vessels	Disability, loss of Smell	
APANGA 1/2 Anguli	2	Face	Lateral corner of Eyex	Blood vessels	Disability, Blindness	
AVARTA 1/2 Anguli	2	Face	Above Eyebrows on lateral side	Joint	Disability, Blindness	
SHANKHA 2 Anguli	2	Head	Temple, between Ear and Apanga	Bone	Sudden death	Control of large Intestine
UTKSHEPA 1/2 Anguli	2	Head	Above Shankha Marma	Ligament	Vishalyaghna (Death occurs if foreign body is removed}	Control of large Intestine

NAME (Extent in Finger Units)	No.	Site	Location	Composition	Effects of Severe Injury	Importance in Treatment
STHAPANI ½ Anguli	1	Head	In between the the center of Eyebrows	Blood vessel	Vishalyaghna	Control of mind and nerves by oil application
SHRINGATAKANI 4 Anguli	4	Head	Soft palate	Blood	Sudden death	Control of Nerves
SIMANTA	5	Head	On the joints of skull bones	Joint	Slow death	Control of Nerves
ADHIPATI ½ Anguli	1	Head	Center of Occiput	Joint	Sudden death	Control of Mind and Nerves

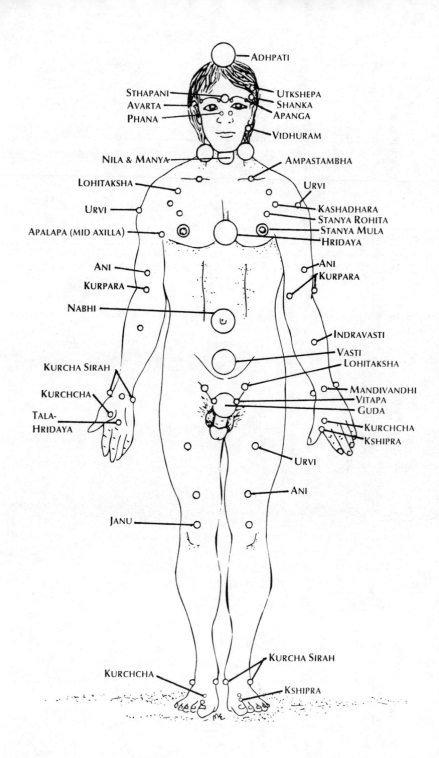

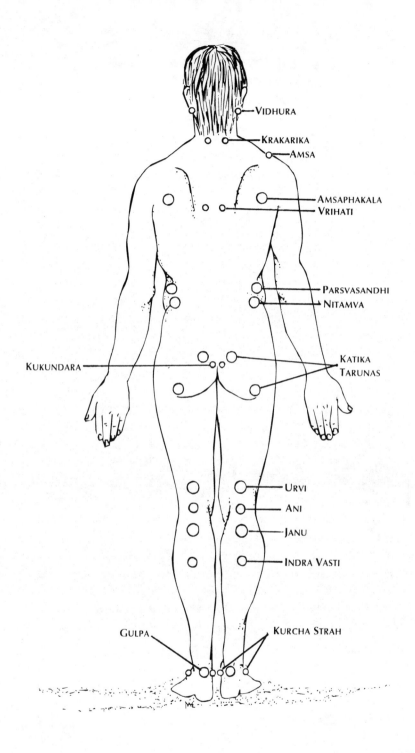

VIDHURA

KRAKARIKA

AMSA

AMSAPHAKALA
VRIHATI

PARSVASANDHI
NITAMVA

KUKUNDARA

KATIKA
TARUNAS

URVI

ANI

JANU

INDRA VASTI

GULPA

KURCHA STRAH

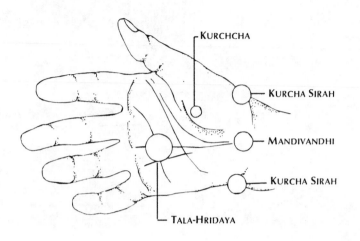

KURCHCHA

KURCHA SIRAH

MANDIVANDHI

KURCHA SIRAH

TALA-HRIDAYA

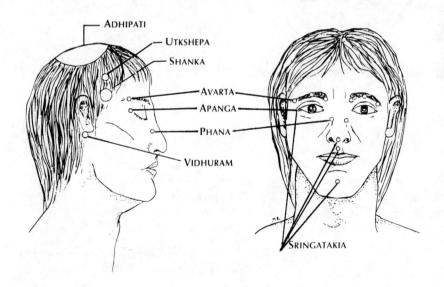

ADHIPATI

UTKSHEPA

SHANKA

AVARTA

APANGA

PHANA

VIDHURAM

SRINGATAKIA

11
TREATMENT OF
THE CHANNEL SYSTEMS

Much of Ayurvedic diagnosis and treatment follows the channel systems (Srotas), as these cover all the functions of the body. They provide us a means of gauging not only the nature but the level of the disease. Below are outlined the main factors in their treatment.

RESPIRATORY SYSTEM (Pranavaha Srotas)

The combined heart and lung apparatus is the main seat of this system. Although it can be equated with the respiratory system, this is not entirely accurate. Its action extends to the brain and its centers, which is the chief site of the life-force or Prana.

Causes of vitiation or disturbance are malnutrition, wasting diseases, excessive physical exercise, dehydration, polluted air, and dust, as well as an excess of Vata or Kapha. Signs of vitiation are rapid, shallow, abnormal, disturbed, or painful respiration. Additional symptoms are cough, wheezing, discoloration due to dyspnea, and various inflammatory conditions of the lungs and upper respiratory tract.

Treatment is according to the treatment of asthma. One should consider the prominence of Vata and Kapha while treating these disorders. For all kinds of inflammatory conditions, Pitta must be treated.

Sthapani Marma, the point which lies between the eyebrows, and Talahridaya Marmas, the point at the center of both the palms of the hand and soles of feet, should be massaged with warm oils to the stimulate lung and heart. In particular, Dhara Tail should be applied on Sthapani Marma.

Alternate nostril breathing should be done regularly to increase the strength of the heart-lung system. As the mind is related to Vata, when respiratory diseases arise due to disturbed mind and emotions, the practice of meditation is essential.

WATER METABOLISM SYSTEM (Udakavasha Srotas)

The hard and soft palates in the mouth are the main seats of this system. It is damaged by excess drinking of alcohol and other liquids, by not taking proper fluids, by eating too many dry food substances, working in heat, by fright, and by indigestion. Excess salt and excessive thirst are additional factors. Signs of vitiation are dryness of the mouth, constant thirst, retention of fluid in various organs as in pleurisy, ascites, the formation of tumors with fluid inside, and generalized edema.

This system is treated along the line of treatment for excessive thirst (Trishna). In these diseases, Vata is very important. If too much fluid has accumulated in any organ or if there is edema, then salt restriction and potassium supplementation should be carried out. Diuretic herbs like punarnava, gokshura, and lemon grass are important.

Treating Basti Marma, the point between the umbilicus and pubic region which controls Kapha, is important, as water is the chief element of Kapha. Along with this, treating Urvi Marma in the mid-upper arm and mid-thigh region gives excellent results.

DIGESTIVE SYSTEM (Annavaha Srotas)

The esophagus and stomach are the chief sites of this system. It is damaged by eating junk food, fast food, improper food, and food which is not properly cooked, overcooked, or unwholesome food having an improper mixture of substances, as well as by any irregular eating habits. Signs of vitiation are indigestion, gas formation, pain in the gastric region or burning sensation, sensation of vomiting, and on rare occasions vomiting with blood.

Most disorders of the digestive system originate due to disturbance in Jatharagni or the digestive fire. Hence correction of the digestive fire is the key to treating the diseases of this system. Herbs like Trikatu (ginger, black pepper, and long pepper), chitrak, and cayenne are good for this purpose. High Pitta conditions like hyperacidity and ulcers should be treated with demulcent herbs like shatavari, amalaki, and licorice, and bland food like milk and mung beans.

For stimulating digestion through Marma points, the four Indra Basti Marmas, two on the mid-lower arm and two at the mid-calf region, should be used. These points can be massaged by different medicated oils.

CIRCULATORY SYSTEM (Rasavaha Srotas)
(Lymphatic portion)

The heart and blood vessels are the main seat of this system. Through this system, the absorbed portion of food circulates in the body along with the lymph and blood and supplies all the nutrients to the tissues. Hence if food is not digested properly due to low digestive fire and Ama or toxins are formed, this system gets disturbed. Excess eating and drinking and too much stress and strain are other factors. All the abnormalities of the SA node in the heart, which disturb the circulation, and other heart conditions including enlargement of the heart also damage this system.

Signs of vitiation are disinclination for food, anorexia, bad taste in the mouth, impotence, wasting away of body tissues, loss of gastric fire, premature formation of wrinkles, and premature graying of the hair. Along with these signs, palpitations, bradycardia, or tachycardia should be considered.

While treating the lymphatic system, proper attention must be given to maintaining its optimal circulation in the body. In Naturopathy a special kind of massage is used to improve the circulation of lymph that is called "lymph drainage massage." In the front of the body, one should massage on the neck down to the clavicle and sternum. As the armpits and groins contain many lymph nodes, proper attention must be paid to these areas. On the abdomen, circular massage should be done.

As the lymph is Kapha in nature, a general anti-Kapha therapy is often useful while treating this system. The digestive fire should be maintained in good order as described under Annavaha Srotas.

CIRCULATORY SYSTEM (Raktavaha Srotas) (Blood or Hemoglobin portion)

The liver and spleen are the main organs of this system. Causes of vitiation are food that is very spicy or hot, and that causes a burning sensation. This increases Pitta and vitiates blood. Many herbs having a hot energy, like cayenne, can vitiate the blood if not used properly. Signs of vitiation are skin disorders like acne and skin rashes, bleeding from urine or feces, bleeding under the skin, inflammation of the rectum, and stomatitis. Enlargement of liver and spleen, abscesses, tumors, bluish-black spots on the skin, jaundice, and leucoderma are additional factors.

Palliation of Pitta and the use of alterative or blood-cleansing herbs like manjishta, turmeric, or burdock are the most important part of the treatment. Ayuredic coral oxide (Prawal Bhasma) and pearl oxide (Moti Bhasma), and bitter purgatives like rhubarb root are also helpful. When conditions like anemia exist, diet and herbs to increase the blood like green vegetables and Suvarna Makshika (a purified iron compound) should be given.

For stimulating the blood system, massage to certain Marma points is a must, especially Hridaya Marma. The twelve Marma points in the region of the throat — the eight Sira Matruka Marmas on both sides of the neck, the two Nila, and two Manya Marmas — should also be considered.

MUSCULAR SYSTEM (Mamsava Srotas)

The muscles and skin are the main sites of this system. Causes of vitiation are over-consumption of heavy, oily, and greasy food, and sleeping after eating. Kapha is the main Dosha connected to this system. All diseases arising out of the muscles like various tumors, piles, warts, sloughing of flesh, and gangrene in the muscle, are signs of its vitiation. Muscular pain is due to high Vata and muscular inflammation due to high Pitta.

For treating muscular pain, rubefacient herbs which increase blood circulation and remove pain like mustard and cinnamon should be used if the pain is due to injury and congestion. If the pain is due to high Vata, then anti-Vata tonifying herbs like shatavari and oils prepared from it like Narayan oil should be used. If the pain is due to Vata which is increased due to obstruction, then oils like Vishgarbha should be used. For treating other disorders like tumors etc., the digestive fire of the muscle tissue (Mamsavaha Agni) should be improved by using herbs like ashwagandha. If it is not possible to eliminate muscle tumors by these means then Agnikarma, cauterization by using probes of gold, copper or iron should be used, or cauterization by alkalies prepared out of plants.

ADIPOSE SYSTEM (Medovaha Srotas)

The fat around the kidneys and omentum in the abdomen are the main sites of this system. Excessive consumption of fatty substances, lack of exercise, and over-indulgence in wine can disturb this system. Excessive eating of sweet, salty, and sour foods, dairy products, sugar, and beef and meat consumption vitiates this system. Obesity and diseases arising out of obesity like hypertension, heart disease, diabetes, and arthritis are the chief signs of diseases of this system. Lipomas or fatty tumors and conditions of arteriosclerosis are also important.

The main factor in treating this system is to normalize the metabolism of this adipose tissue. For this herbs like guggul, myrrh, and rasna should be used in combinations with those like cyperus, chitrak, or black pepper. Deep massage work with dry powder of talcum or calamus or with oils which are hot like mustard should be done. Kapha is closely linked with adipose tissue. Hence it can also be good to give Vamana or herb-induced emesis.

In obese patients, Guda Marma should be massaged. If this is tender, then it should be considered as an indication of some obstruction in the system. At such times therapeutic vomiting is helpful to get rid of excess Kapha obstructing the channels.

SKELETAL SYSTEM (Asthivaha Srotas)

Adipose tissue around bones and buttocks are the main sites. The bones and Vata are closely related. This means that if the colon, the chief site of Vata, gets disturbed, or if Vata otherwise gets disturbed, then this system becomes vitiated. Similarly, external injuries causing fractures, violent movements of the body, and Vata-increasing diet can disturb this system. Pain in the bones, hypertrophy or atrophy of bones, discoloration and other pathological conditions of the hair and nails, and various tumors of the bones indicate diseases of this system.

In treatment, Vata should be controlled by stimulating Sthapani and Adhipati Marmas. For correcting the disturbance in the colon, Shankha Marma in the temples and Utkshepa Marma just below it should be massaged. Substances which contain natural calcium, like oyster shells or sesame seeds, are good to treat the bones. Enemas with sesame oil or those containing milk, ghee and nutritive herbs like ashwagandha and shatavari are extremely good.

NERVOUS SYSTEM (Majjavaha Srotas)

The long bones and joints are the main sites of this system. The main cause of its vitiation is injury to the skull, vertebral column, and other long bones, which crushes the marrow. Infections, high fevers, and improper food habits that increase Vata also tend to disturb this system. Pain in the joints, giddiness, fainting, lack of coordination in movement, paralysis or paresis of the muscles, and wrong reception of sensations of touch and temperature are important signs of diseases of this system.

High Vata and high Pitta can disturb this system. As Pitta accumulates in the small intestine, through controlling this organ one can also control excess Pitta in the nervous system. Nervine stimulants like calamus and sedatives like gotu kola, jatamansi, and shankhapushpi are primary for treating this system. Similarly the five Simanta Marmas situated in the cranial sutures and the four Sringataka Marmas should be treated appropriately. Sthapani and Adhipati Marmas treated by Shirodhara (dripping of medicated oil) is good for disorders like insomnia, loss of sensory function, and paralysis. Enema treatment with oily and tonifying enemas also helps.

REPRODUCTIVE SYSTEM (SHUKRAVAHA SROTAS)

In men, the testes and penis are the chief sites of this system (for women see the Menstrual System). Untimely sexual intercourse or unnatural sex acts, suppression of the sexual urge, excessive sexual indulgence, and bad effects of various surgical procedures are behind the various diseases of this system. Owing to excessive sexual indulgence Ojas becomes depleted. This reduces longevity and increases Vata, which can cause various Vata disorders like tuberculosis, consumption, or other wasting disorders (including the modern disease of AIDS). Permanent sterility or impotency can also result. Diseases like enlargement of the prostate and hydrocele are included under this system.

In cases of impotence, food and herbs that increase the reproductive fluids should be given. For this, rejuvenative (Rasayana) and invigorating (Vajikarana) herbs play an important part, like ashwagandha, kapikacchu, and shatavari. Control of Apana Vayu is also essential. For this Guda Marma and Kukundara Marma should be treated with oil massage.

URINARY SYSTEM (MUTRAVAHA SROTAS)

The large intestine and urinary bladder are the main sites of this system. It is damaged by such factors as excessive or insufficient drinking of water, excessive heat and dry climate, constantly working near fire, or toxic substances. Signs of its damage are painful urination, burning urination, lack of urination, urinary tract infections, or stones in the urinary system.

Treatment is mainly through diuretic (urination promoting) herbs, of which there are many. Most frequently used in Ayurveda are punarnava and gokshura. In inflammatory conditions, anti-Pitta herbs should be used. Katika, Taruna, and Kukundar Marma along with Basti Marma points should be massaged. This stimulates all the urinary organs in a beneficial manner.

EXCRETORY SYSTEM (PURISHAVAHA SROTAS)

The rectum and anal canal are the chief sites of this system. It is damaged by suppression of the urge to defecate, by eating food that has too much roughage, or food which is pre-digested and has too little roughage. When the digestive power is weak this system also gets vitiated. Signs of its improper functioning are diarrhea, constipation, dysentery, pain in the colon, colitis, blood in the stool, and hemorrhoids.

Treatment varies according to the condition. In cases of diarrhea, before giving astringent herbs to bind the stool make sure that any toxins in the colon have first been flushed out. Then one can use astringents like kutaj. In amoebic dysentery, excess Kapha should be treated along with high Vata by giving sesame oil enemas. For constipation, the herbal formula Triphala can be used for mild constipation, while for more severe constipation purgatives like castor oil or senna can be used. Krikatika and Sandhi Marma are important points to massage for this system.

SWEAT SYSTEM (SWEDAVAHA SROTAS)

The origin of this system is in the adipose tissue and the pores on the skin. It is damaged by overexposure to the elements (wind, cold, or heat) and overexercise. Anger or fear, the eating of hot and spicy food, excess or insufficient drinking of water, and drinking of wine are additional vitiating factors. Signs of its vitiation are excess or deficient sweating, skin rashes, or skin diseases.

Treatment is mainly through diaphoretic (sweat-promoting) herbs and through Oleation (Snehana) and Sudation (Swedana) therapies. Diaphoretics like cinnamon increase sweating, while astringents like lodhra or alum root counter excess sweating.

MENSTRUAL SYSTEM (ARTAVAVAHA SROTAS)

The uterus and fallopian tubes are the main sites of this system. Increase of Pitta and Vata primarily cause the disoders of the system such as premenstrual tension (P.M.S.), discomfort and pain during menstruation (dysmenorrhea), absence of menstruation (amenorrhoea), excessive bleeding during menstruation (menorrhagia), and various discomforts at the time of menopause.

In treating this system, Apana Vayu, the downward moving air, is important. Hence the same Marma points as given for the treatment of the urinary system should be considered. Emmenagogue (menstruation-promoting) herbs like saffron, turmeric, or motherwort should be used when needed. For symptoms due to stress and strain, sedatives like valerian or jatamansi should be used.

LACTATION SYSTEM (STANYAVAHA SROTAS)

The breasts and nipples are the main sites of this system, which is active during the period of lactation after childbirth. Improper care of the breasts during pregnancy and food that increases Vata and Kapha disturbs this system. Signs of vitiation are deficient milk supply, impure milk, breast tumors, or abscesses.

For increasing the quantity of milk, galactagogue herbs like shatavari, licorice, and sesame seeds are good. For removing the bad qualities of milk due to excess Doshas, cyperus, fennel, dill, or dandelion are good.

12
YOGA
AND AYURVEDA

A person who studies one branch of learning only cannot arrive at proper conclusions. Therefore, a physician should strive to learn as many related sciences as possible. — *Sushruta*

At present there are many alternative systems of medicine engaged in health maintenance and the treatment of disease. Yet it is surprising that although the human body is everywhere the same, each medical science approaches it in different ways. The science of acupuncture tries to understand the human body in terms of the principles of Yin and Yang, while the Unani system considers it to be composed of four humors or energies. Both the sciences of Yoga and Ayurveda have evolved from the same philosophy, culture, and country. They look at the human being from the same holistic angle. Both are special sciences of antiquity.

Ayurveda is the science of life or longevity. Yoga is the science of linking the individual self with the universal Self. Yoga tries to expand the narrow constricted egoistic personality to the all-pervasive, eternal, and blissful state of reality. Both sciences aim at developing the physical, mental, intellectual, emotional, and spiritual levels of the human being.

According to Ayurveda, the human being is composed of body, senses, mind, and spirit. Thus Ayurveda considers life a psycho-spiritual as well as a somatic (physical) phenomenon. Basically it aims at ending all suffering and maintaining health, so that every individual can achieve all four goals of life — honor, wealth, enjoyment, and liberation (Dharma, Artha, Kama, and Moksha). The aim of Yoga is mainly to achieve the psycho-spiritual goal of life or liberation, but it has not neglected the importance of maintaining health in the process of pursuing it.

Purity of body, mind, and speech is essential for the ultimate welfare of the human being. Three basic texts have been written, one on each of them. Many scholars believe that the same author, under different names, has written these, that the Patanjali of the Yoga text and of the grammatical text is the same as the Charaka of the Ayurvedic text. These three books are:

- *The Yoga Sutras* of Patanjali — the classical work on the science of Yoga for purification of mind and realization of the Self
- *The Mahabhashya* of Patanjali — for purification of speech, an important work on grammar and speech, the main commentary on Panini's grammar
- *The Charaka Samhita* of Charaka — for purification of the physical body, the main text of Ayurveda

FUNDAMENTAL PRINCIPLES

Both Ayurveda and Yoga share the same fundamental principles and look at the anatomy, physiology, and treatment of the human body in the same manner. As the basis of understanding the human body is the same for both sciences, it is essential that anyone intending to study either one of them should learn the other as well. Both of these ancient sciences are Indian in origin and accept common principles from the Sankhya system of philosophy. Yoga and Ayurveda originate as part of the greater system of Vedic science passed on from the ancient seers, the rishis of the Himalayas.

Both Ayurveda and Yoga are based upon the principles of the three Gunas (Sattva, Rajas, and Tamas) and the theory of the five great elements. They both use the humor-tissue-waste material theory (Dosha-Dhatu-Mala) for understanding the workings of the body, and the taste-energy-post-digestive effect concept (Rasa-Virya-Vipaka) for understanding the use of foods and medicines. Initially both these sciences had eight branches, the "eightfold" paths of Ashtanga Yoga and Ashtanga Ayurveda.

Ayurveda is the science of healthy living. Hence Ayurveda explains in detail the signs of longevity. Some Yoga textbooks also describe these same signs and symptoms as well.

ANATOMY AND PHYSIOLOGY

Yoga textbooks advise us to study anatomy according to Ayurveda, because unless one knows anatomy adequately, Yogic purificatory practices cannot be properly performed. On the other hand, Ayurvedic textbooks, while explaining anatomy, have pointed out that this study is for practitioners of Yoga as well as physicians. For explaining human anatomy both sciences employ the same terminology of blood vessels (Shira), nerves (Dhamanya), tissues (Dhatus), and so on.

The three Doshas or biological humors are the three energy principles which govern all physiological activities in the body. The tissues or

Dhatus (plasma, blood, muscle, fat, bone, nervous, and reproductive tissues) provide stability to the body and the Malas (urine, feces, and sweat) are waste products. These are the three important constituents of the human body. Both sciences recognize these basic constituents and stress that their equilibrium is essential for health.

Ayurveda has accepted the concept of Agni-Soma emphasized in Yogic texts. These two principles dominate all activities in the universe and in the human being. In the body, the right side is Sun-Agni dominant, while the left side is Moon-Soma dominant. This principle has been used for advising only right or left nostril breathing for certain diseases.

Vata, the principal energy of movement in the body, has a close relationship with Agni, the power of digestion. Hence both sciences explain that control of Vata is essential for controlling the power of digestion.

That health of the body depends upon the equilibrium of the humors, tissues and waste-materials is explained in the *Hatha Yoga Pradipika*[1], the most important Hatha Yoga text. Similarly, Ayurveda accepts certain Yoga principles, most importantly that health of the body is dependent on health and balance of the mind. The mind is inherently unstable like mercury and hence can be easily agitated and disturbed. It is kept calm and under control by restraining emotions like anger, fear, and greed, a practice which is beneficial for maintaining health. Regular practice of Pranayama or yogic breathing is helpful for gaining control over the mind. Also there is a correlation between mind and Vata. A healthy mind can control Vata, and control over Vata keeps the mind in control. Thus mind and Vata are mutually related and their interaction can be helpful or harmful depending on how we allow it to function. This concept is prominent in both sciences.

Ayurveda holds that health practices and therapies should always be adopted in a step-by-step manner. Similarly the *Hatha Yoga Pradipika* states that postures and Pranayama should be undertaken gradually. Both systems aim at gradual and natural deep internal changes, not at radical, forced, superficial, and symptomatic results.

For maintenance of health, both sciences explain a similar beneficial diet, life-style, and ethical regimen. While explaining different exercises, Sushruta gives importance to Yogic postures. Both sciences have accepted that control over the sense organs is essential for the preservation of health.

TREATMENT

Both Yoga and Ayurveda advocate the use of herbs, food, and the chanting of mantras for physical and mental health. Ayurveda stresses the use of herbs and medicines for curing diseases, but Yoga also advises the use of herbs for purification of the mind. For treating psychological disorders as well as physical diseases, Ayurveda has its psychological and spiritual (Sattvavajaya) therapy. This aims at increasing the clear or Sattvic quality of mind and basically comes from the science of Yoga. Yogic procedures like Pranayama are particularly useful in this regard.

Almost all Yoga textbooks use the Ayurvedic terminology of the Doshas, the digestive fire, and so on for explaining the effects of postures and Pranayama. They also follow the Ayurvedic nomenclature for diseases.[2] It has been clearly stated that when limitations to Ayurvedic treatment are observed, one should consult a Yoga teacher. Similarly, when side effects of improperly done Yoga practices occur they should be treated by Ayurvedic remedies.

The Purification Practices of Ayurveda and Yoga

When the conversion of food takes place, many waste products are formed. Similarly, owing to wrong eating habits or an impaired digestive process, toxic substances are formed in the body. If these toxins are not eliminated properly, diseases are formed. For maintenance of proper health, elimination of waste products at the proper time is essential. Both sciences have given equal importance to this principle. Their purification practices, Ayurvedic Pancha Karma and Yogic Shuddhi Kriyas, are based on this principle. *Hatha Yoga Pradipika* has even explained that Ayurvedic oleation and sudation should be done prior to Yogic purification practices and that Ayurvedic enemas and nasal medications (Basti and Nasya) should be done every day.

Rejuvenation

To gain the maximum benefits of Rasayana or rejuvenation treatment, every person must follow an ethical regimen. The description of Yama and Niyama in Yoga, the ethical observances and disciplines necessary for the right practice of Yoga, are very similar to ethical regimen in Ayurveda. Yoga has explained that persons who follow the rules of Yama and Niyama derive the maximum benefits of Yoga practices. The construction of the Yoga chamber for Yoga practices is very similar to the construction of the special chamber (Trigarbha Kuti) for Kutipraveshika Rasayana.

Liberation

Charaka has explained the law of similarity between the universe and man. The universe is the macrocosm, while man is the microcosm. The realization that the entire universe and the individual are one and the same is called "Satya-buddhi," which literally means "the ascertainment of truth."

Satya-buddhi is the state of realization of the ultimate reality. It eliminates all miseries and leads to liberation (Moksha). Charaka has explained that ego (selfhood or mineness) is the cause of all miseries. The moment that the ascertainment of truth (Satya-buddhi) emerges, the soul or Atman transcends the ego and all worldly miseries end. It has also been explained that action (pravritti) which is initiated by Karma (the results of past actions) is the root cause of all miseries. Satya-buddhi transcends all karmas and affords freedom from action (nivritti). This freedom from action or state of inaction is considered to be the highest achievement. The state of inaction and ultimate realization (Moksha) are the same. Thus Charaka describes the highest quality of Yogic achievement or knowledge of ultimate truth and he also teaches how to achieve it.

Yogic science has explained that in order to achieve liberation, one has to proceed from the physical sheath (Annamaya Kosha) to the Pranic or breath sheath (Pranamaya Kosha), then to the mental sheath (Manomaya Kosha), and from there to the wisdom sheath (Vijñanamaya Kosha), and finally to the bliss sheath (Anandamaya Kosha). By different Yoga procedures, one can transcend these sheaths and ultimately achieve liberation or the state of pure consciousness (Purusha).

In summary, Yoga and Ayurveda are in all respects allied as sister sciences. Ayurveda envisages the total welfare of man, material and spiritual, while Yoga specifically ensures his psycho-spiritual development. In view of the fundamental unity of these two ancient spiritual sciences, it appears useful to revive and develop them together to construct a total and holistic positive health science for the benefit of humanity as a whole.

DIFFERENT METHODS OF YOGA

We have seen that Yoga is the science which helps to firmly unite the physical body with the spiritual being. It is also a practice to obtain control of one's latent powers. Many methods have been described to achieve this goal. In this chapter, we shall discuss them briefly.

Patanjali's Ashtanga Yoga

This is perhaps the classical system of Yoga and aspects of it are found in most Yoga systems. It is also recognized within the field of Ayurveda. It consists of eight limbs or portions (ashtanga).

YAMA — These are ten rules which every Yoga practitioner should follow. They are non-violence, truthfulness, non-stealing, control of sexual energy, forbearance or forgiveness, fortitude, mercy, straightforwardness, purity, and moderation in diet.

NIYAMA — These are the ten restrictions of self-discipline, contentment, faith, charity, good company, modesty, control of the mind, chanting of mantras, devotion to God, and observation of vows.

ASANA — means different postures. In all, eighty-four varieties have been described. It must always be remembered that postures are not acrobatic exercises. All Yoga postures require slow contraction and slow relaxation, with concentration on breathing.

PRANAYAMA — is the breathing technique for controlling the life-force or Prana.

PRATYAHARA — is a method for withdrawal of the mind from the senses, or not to be attached to the objects of enjoyment through the senses.

DHARANA — means focusing the mind for concentration.

DHYANA — means meditation with concentration.

SAMADHI — means integration of the perceiver and the perceived through continuous concentrated meditation.

Hatha Yoga

Hatha Yoga is perhaps the most well-known Yoga practice in the Western world. Of Yoga practices it is the most directly related to the physical body, though it has much that goes beyond it as well. The term Hatha is composed of two syllables "Ha" meaning the Sun or solar principle and "Tha" meaning the Moon or lunar principle. Our body is divided into two principles. The right side is Sun-dominant while the left is Moon-dominant. Health is maintained only when there is equilibrium between both parts. With the help of Hatha Yoga one can achieve this equilibrium. For this Hatha Yoga prscribes the first five principles described in Ashtanga Yoga. In addition it also gives much emphasis to six special purificatory procedures.

Karma Yoga

Karma Yoga means service (Seva) or selfless work, action done with an attitude of detachment for the fruits of the action. All misery and pain comes from attachment. If such selfless work is done one gains freedom from all misery and pain.

Bhakti Yoga

This teaches how to worship and pray to God with love and affection. With this type of Yoga, man learns to gain control over emotional instabilities and ultimately love the entire world.

Jñana Yoga

This form of Yoga teaches the process of right reasoning and inquiry leading to thought-free meditation. With this practice one learns with acuity of mind how to approach the ultimate truth.

Raja Yoga

This is the process through which one can control the mind. By controlling the mind, one can learn a practical and easy approach to reach higher states of consciousness. It is mainly based on the inner aspects (antaranga) of Patanjali's Ashtanga Yoga system which comprise concentration, meditation, and realization (Dharana, Dhyana, and Samadhi).

Kundalini Yoga and Tantra

Kundalini Yoga teaches how to gain control over the dormant power of the Kundalini or psychic energy of transformation. Kundalini dwells at the base of the spine where the three psychic nerves (Ida, Pingala, and Sushumna) come together. These three are comparable to the right and left sympathetic chains and the spinal cord. The Kundalini awakening is done gradually from the sacral plexus (Muladhara Chakra) to the lumbar plexus (Svadhisthana Chakra) to the celiac plexus (Manipura Chakras), the cardic plexus (Anahata Chakra), the pulmonary plexus (Vishuddha Chakra), the cervical plexus (Ajña Chakra) and finally, when the Kundalini ascends to Sahasrara (hypothalamus) one gains control over the autonomic nervous system and reaches a stage of spiritual bliss.

Kundalini is emphasized in various Tantric practices, which include a number of yogic approaches like Mantra Yoga, Japa Yoga, Laya Yoga (the Yoga of the sound current). These methods are used for spiritual purposes or for gaining occult powers.

YOGA POSTURES FOR DIFFERENT CONSTITUTIONS

A person who wishes to practice Hatha Yoga should avoid over-eating, overexertion, too much talking, excess public contact, and changeability of mind. Then if one practices Yoga postures, Pranayama and yogic purification practices, along with Yama and Niyama, one will obtain all the benefits of Yoga like slimness of body, lustre of the face, clearness of voice, brightness of the eyes, freedom from disease, control over sexual energy, good digestive power, and purification of all the Nadis or nerves.

Main Yoga Postures for Vata Constitution

The simple sitting poses described below are very useful for Vata constitutions.

SUKHASANA OR EASY POSTURE — Sit on a mat with the legs stretched out in front. Then bend the right leg at the knee and place the right foot under the left thigh by using your hand if required. Now bend the left leg and place the left foot under your right leg. Keep the vertebral column or spine erect. Extend both arms so that the wrists rest on the knees with palms turned upwards.

SIDDHASANA — Sit on a mat with the legs stretched out in front. Then bend the right leg at the knee and place the heal of the foot under the perineum. Now bend the left leg and bring the left heel against the pubic bone. Place both hands as in Sukhasana.

PADMASANA OR LOTUS POSTURE — First sit on the mat with the legs stretched out in front. Then with the help of the hands bring the right foot to rest on the left thigh, close to the hip joint, with the sole of the foot turned upwards and the left heel near the middle of the abdomen. Then bend the left foot and bring the left foot onto the right thigh by crossing it over the right leg. Keep the spine erect and close the eyes. Both the hands should be kept as in Sukhasana.

Main Yoga Postures for Pitta Constitution

BHUJANGASANA OR THE COBRA POSE — Lie face down on the mat. Keep the legs together, chin touching the ground and the soles of the feet facing up. Keep the arms bent near the body, so the palms touch the ground near the shoulder, and keep the arms bent at the elbow. Raise the head slowly first and then the upper portion of the body until the navel area is about to lift above the ground. During this time no pressure should be placed on the hands. After maintaining this position for some time, return to the lying-down position.

VIPARITAKARINI — Lie flat on your back with legs stretched out and both hands near the body. Keeping the knees stiff, try slowly to raise both legs at an angle of forty-five degrees. Keep the position for some time, then return to normal position.

SARVANGASANA OR SHOULDER STAND — Lie flat on your back with legs stretched out. Then first come to the position of Viparitakarini. Raise the legs further up to a ninety degree angle. Now raise the buttocks and the trunk as well, taking support of the arms and elbows, without lifting the head. Rest the elbows on the ground firmly and support the back with both palms. Straighten the trunk with the hands till the chin is well set in at the suprasternal notch. Maintain this position and then slowly return to normal.

HALASANA OR PLOUGH POSE — Raise the legs till they are ninety degrees, as in the shoulder stand. Then slowly swing them over your head until the toes of the legs touch the ground. Keep the knees stiff and the palms of your hands flat on the floor, with the arms stretched. Maintain this position and then slowly return to normal position.

Main Postures for Kapha Constitution

PASCHIMOTASANA — Sit on the mat with legs stretched out in front. Bend the trunk slowly and try to hook your fingers into the big toes of both feet. Then slowly bend the back further forward so that the trunk is stretched along the thighs and the face rests on the knees. Maintain and then return to normal position.

SIX YOGIC PURIFICATION PRACTICES

Patanjali has described six purificatory actions (Shuddhi Kriyas) which are useful for purifying the body. They are: 1) Kapalabhati, 2) Neti, 3) Dhouti, 4) Nauli, 5) Trataka, and 6) Basti. In the section on Pranayama, we will discuss the technique of Kapalabhati. In this chapter we will discuss the remaining five practices.

Neti — Nasal Cleansing

Four types of Neti or nasal cleansing are in general practice: Jala Neti, water cleansing; Sutra Neti, cleansing with a cloth; Dugha Neti, cleansing with milk; and Ghrita Neti, cleansing with ghee or clarified butter.

WATER CLEANSING OR JALA NETI — Add about half a teaspoon of salt to a Neti pot which is full of lukewarm water. Hold the pot in the right hand. Insert the nozzle of the pot into the right nostril. Keep the mouth open to allow free breathing through the mouth.

Tilt the head first slightly backwards, then forward and sideways to the left so that the water from the pot enters the right nostril and comes out through the left by the force of gravity. Let it flow till the pot is empty. Should there be congestion that prevents the flow of water, allow some time to elapse and the passage may open, or tilt the head down and let the water flow out the same nostril and try again.

Repeat the same process on the left side. When the process is complete, take out the remaining water from the nasal passage by gently forced exhalations through the nostrils. Generally it is better to exhale through both nostrils, as this helps regulate the pressure in the head. In this cleansing process mucus and other impurities will be discharged into the water.

By slightly bending the head back, the water goes to the mouth and can be swallowed after washing the passage as described above. This is called "Usah Pana," which can be practiced every morning before sunrise and has beneficial effects.

Please note that the amount of salt can be adjusted according to the individual. Too much salt may cause a burning sensation, too little can irritate the mucous membranes. The temperature of the water can also be adjusted; usually slightly warm is good, not hot or cold. Some people may find tap water, which is chlorinated, to be irritating. They should use spring or distilled water. Herbal decoctions can also be used instead of water for more specific therapeutic purposes.

SUTRA NETI OR RUBBER CATHETER NETI — Insert the blunt end of a thin soft rubber catheter from the front horizontally into the right nostril. The catheter should be previously lubricated with sesame or some other oil.

Push it along the floor of the nose until the tip is felt in the back of the throat. Insert the right index and the middle fingers through the mouth and catch the tip of the catheter at the back of the throat. Pull it out through the mouth and gently massage the nasal passage by catching the two ends of the tube. Remove the catheter through the nose. Repeat the same procedure on the left side after lubricating the catheter again.

This process requires some skill and should not be done unless one is proficient at Jala Neti. It may cause nausea or vomiting in some people and should be done with care.

DUGHA NETI AND GHRITA NETI — The procedure for these is the same as for Jala Neti, only instead of water, milk and ghee are used. Medicated ghees and oils and herbal decoctions in milk can also be used in this manner.

Dhouti — Cleansing the Stomach

This procedure cleanses the intestinal tract down to the stomach. Three types of Dhouti will be explained: Jala Dhouti or Vamana Dhouti, water cleansing; Vastra Dhouti, cleansing with a cloth; and Danda Dhouti, cleansing with a tube. While we mention the procedure for doing the forms of Dhouti that require swallowing a cloth or rubber tube, we do not recommend trying them on your own. They should be done only by the careful and experienced instruction of a competent Yoga teacher. Some people have harmed themselves by attempting to do these practices without the right guidance.

JALA DHOUTI OR VAMANA DHOUTI, WATER CLEANSING — Sit on the heels and drink lukewarm saline water until you can take no more or until there is a sensation of vomiting. Churn the stomach by twisting exercise.

Stand with feet together and bend forward, forming an angle of about ninety degrees, and vomit. If you cannot vomit easily, tickle the back of the throat so that with the sensation of vomiting all the water will be vomited out.

This is essentially the same practice as Vamana or emetic therapy in Ayurveda. Similar herbal substances can be used to increase its therapeutic effectiveness. It can be a helpful daily practice done early in the morning to remove excess Kapha.

VASTRA DHOUTI, CLEANSING WITH A CLOTH — Take a very soft cloth having four fingers breadth and seven meters length. Put it into water or milk so that it becomes soft. Then it is slowly swallowed until it reaches the stomach.

After a short time, slowly bring out the cloth while exhaling, without using any force. This procedure is called Vastra Dhouti. During swallowing or while taking out the cloth, if it sticks at one place drink some water to release the spasm.

Swallowing the cloth may cause some nausea or vomiting reflex. It should not be done by those with sensitive or nervous stomachs, nor should it be attempted by those who have not first mastered the Jala Dhouti or water cleansing. Be sure to use a cloth made of natural fibers like cotton and one that does not have any harmful dyes.

DANDA DHOUTI — Drink lukewarm saline water as in Jala Dhouti. Then take a flexible rubber tube (Danda) about one centimeter in diameter and about one meter long. Slowly start to swallow the tube. When it reaches the stomach, bend forward. All the water first swallowed will come out by syphon action.

This method is yet more difficult and should not be done by those who are not proficient in the other two forms of Dhouti.

Nauli

Nauli is an abdominal action in which isolation and rolling manipulation of the abdominal muscles (which form the front wall) is done.

UDDIYANA — Stand with a slight forward bend of the trunk with palms on the thighs, and the feet about a meter apart.

Exhale completely by vigorously contracting the muscles of the abdomen. At this time the chest also gets contracted. Then press the hands against the thighs and at the same time try to tighten the muscles of the neck and shoulder. Then carry out a vigorous mock-inhalation by raising the ribs without actually allowing the air to flow into the lungs. Relax the muscles of the abdomen. Automatically the diaphragm will rise up, producing a concave depression of the abdomen. This is called Uddiyana.

In this condition and when the breath is entirely exhaled, quickly push out and pull in the abdominal muscles alternately. Continue as long as the retention of the breath lasts. Count the number of contractions. This process is called "Agnisara Kriya." It is very useful for increasing the digestive power.

MADHYAMA NAULI — Maintaining Uddiyana, give a forward and downward push to the abdominal point just above the pelvic bone in the mid-line, where the two recti muscles originate. This push brings about the concentration of these muscles which stand out in the center, leaving the other muscles of the abdominal wall in a relaxed condition. This is Madhyama Nauli.

DAKSHINA AND VAMA NAULI — Dakshina means right. For right side Nauli, one has to contract the right rectus muscle, leaving the other muscles including the left rectus relaxed.

Vama means left. For left side Nauli, the opposite procedure should be done.

NAULI CHALANA — After gaining full control over the first three types, rolling of the rectus abdominous muscles clockwise and anti-clockwise is done. This rolling is called Nauli Chalana.

Trataka — Cleansing the Eyes

This procedure for cleansing the eyes can be done simply, safely and effectively on a regular basis by everyone. Sit in any meditative posture comfortably with an erect spine. Arrange a burning candle or ghee lamp with the flame set at the same height as the eyes and at a distance of about three feet. Gaze at the flame without blinking the eyes. Learn to ignore the irritation and watering of the eyes. With practice, the gaze becomes steady, making the mind also steady. Try to relax the eyes in this position. Progress slowly, starting with thirty seconds and increasing the duration by ten seconds per week.

Trataka is a very useful procedure to purify the vision and increase concentration and will power. It improves our visual capacity and can be helpful in treating headaches and nervous problems. A ghee flame gives better results. For this take a ghee lamp or any small metal bowl. Fill it with ghee and add a wick made of cotton (you can take any ball of cotton and stretch and roll it into the size and shape of a wick).

Benefits of Hatha Yoga

The body becomes lean but sturdy, while strength and immunity are increased. The individual becomes very active and energetic. Dullness and distraction (Tamas and Rajas) decrease and clarity (Sattva) increases. Hence the knowledge of ultimate truth is achieved. Many believe that the practice of Pranayama of the Hatha Yoga type balances Prana and Apana and thereby normalizes Vata.[3]

The initial stages of Hatha Yoga serve to reduce the amount of inertia (Tamas) and attachment to the physical body. To aid in this quality, the individual must follow the rules of diet and behavior laid down by this science. One must then concentrate on various postures and Pranayama. After concentrating the mind on rhythmic breathing, one can achieve tranquility of mind and self-realization. Hatha Yoga therefore is not just physical exercise. It is a way of life and leads us through physical, mental, and ethical disciplines to the ultimate truth.

∗ ∗ ∗

PRANAYAMA

"Prana" means breath and "Ayama" means a pause or retention. Hence Pranayama means a pause in the movement of breath. Patanjali describes Pranayama as a pause in inspiration or expiration.

Types of Pranayama

There are four basic types which are based on the nature of the retention.

- Retention after expiration (rechaka), called an outer retention (bahya kumbhaka)
- Retention after inspiration (puraka), called an inner retention (abhyantara kumbhaka)
- Retention made at once
- Retention after many inhalations and exhalations

These last two forms of retention are called "kevala kumbhka." Thus the action of Pranayama consists of four phases:

- Inspiration — Puraka
- Inner retention — Abhyantara Kumbhaka
- Expiration — Rechaka
- Outer retention — Bahya Kumbhaka

Proportion

The beginner should always practice Pranayama with a one-to-two ratio of inhalation and exhalation, that is with exhalation twice the length of inhalation.

After proficiency in this is gained, one should practice with a proportion of inhalation one, internal retention two, exhalation two, and external retention two.

The ideal proportion is inhalation one, internal retention four, exhalation two, and external retention four, but this takes some time to be able to do with ease. In Pranayama there should be no straining to achieve results but a natural deepening of the breath by letting go of strain and tension.

Technique

The person should sit in Padmasana (lotus posture), Siddhasana, or Svastikasana, but any comfortable seated pose can be used. The place should be well ventilated but the draft of air should not come directly on the body. Open air and a calm and quiet place are preferable.

Pranayama should be performed by closing alternate nostrils. For this the right palm is first spread out. The index and middle fingers are turned down. The other two fingers and the thumb remain extended. Now the thumb and extended fingers are placed on the bridge of the nose, the thumb on the right side and the extended fingers on the left. Then alternately extended fingers are used to close right and left nostril for Pranayama.

EIGHT TYPES OF PRANAYAMA

Patanjali has described eight different types of Pranayama; Ujjayi, Kapalabhati, Bhastrika, Suryabhedana, Sitkari, Shitali, Bhramari, and Plavini. We shall briefly discuss these types.

Ujjayi

The meaning of this word is "to pronounce loudly" or "what leads to success and victory." In this type of Pranayama the breath is drawn through both the nostrils. During inhalation, the glottis is to be partially closed, which will produce sound. Retention should then be done with Jalandhara bandha (chin lock) and then both nostrils should be closed. Then exhalation should be done through the left nostril. The proportion between inhalation and exhalation should be one to two and retention should be done until there is no sensation of suffocation.

Kapalabhati

This is also one of the procedures for cleansing the nasal passages in the head. The actual meaning is "what makes the head shine." Strictly speaking it is not a type of Pranayama. The person should sit in the lotus or any comfortable pose because it is a breathing exercise for abdominal and diaphragmatic muscles and the organs in the portion of the umbilicus.

First a forceful exhalation should be done which is a little deeper than ordinary breathing. At this time the front abdominal muscles are suddenly and vigorously contracted. Then inhalation should be performed by simply relaxing the abdominal muscles. In this procedure retention is not to be done. The beginner should start with eleven expulsions in each round. With each expiration a stroke is delivered to the center of the abdomen which thereby helps to spiritually activate the nervous system.

Bhastrika

Bhastrika is characterized by a quick expulsion of the breath producing a sound like a bellow. It differs little from Kapalabhati. There are four varieties of Bhastrika.

The first type starts out with some quick rounds of Kapalabhati. After the last expulsion of Kapalabhati, a very deep inhalation is done followed by internal retention. Then exhalation should be done slowly, followed by external retention. This entire procedure completes one round of Bhastrika.

The only difference between the first and second type is that in the inhalation-internal retention, exhalation-external retention procedure for the second type should be done only with the right nostril.

In the third variety, quick respirations are done through the right nostril, keeping the left closed. After some rounds, the inhalation should be done through the same nostril. Then retention is done and exhalation through the left nostril.

In the fourth variety, quick inhalation through the right nostril and quick retention through the left nostril should be done until one is fatigued. Then the deepest possible inspiration through the right nostril should be done and, after retention, exhalation should be done through the left nostril.

Suryabhedana

In this type of Pranayama, one breathes in through the Sun-dominant right nostril, then retention should be done until there is perspiration, and exhalation is done through the Moon-dominant left nostril. This type of Pranayama increases heat in the body.

Sitkari

Sit in a comfortable posture with an erect spine. First do exhalation from both nostrils. Fold the tongue backwards and press the tip of the tongue by the hard palate, leaving a small opening on either side of the tongue. Carry out inhalation through these side openings. During this time a hissing sound like "sit" is made. After completing inhalation, the tongue should be withdrawn, the mouth closed, and then retention should be performed.

Shitali

This type of Pranayama produces a cooling effect in the body, hence it has been named Shitali, which means "cooling." For practicing this, fold up the sides of the partially protruded tongue so as to form a long narrow tube resembling the beak of a bird. This passage is further narrowed by pressing the lips round the tongue. Take an inhalation and perceive the cooling effect of the air as it passes through the tongue. Then close the mouth and do retention. Exhalation should be done through both nostrils.

Bhramari

In this type of Pranayama, by quick forced inspiration a humming sound like a bee is produced, hence it is called as Bhramari, which means "the buzzing of a bee."

While doing inhalation, the soft palate should be lifted and drawn toward the nasal part of the pharynx. This produces a sound due to the vibration of the soft palate. Then retention should be done as usual. Exhalation requires the same movement of the soft palate again.

Murccha

Murccha means "temporary loss of consciousness." First inhalation should be done. At the end of inhalation, Jalandhara bandha or the chin lock should be done, followed by retention. This position should be maintained as long as possible, so that it produces a sensation leading to loss of awareness.

Plavini

With this type of Pranayama, one can easily "float on the water" for a long time, hence this name has been given to it. Although any person can float on water, with this type of Pranayama he can remain afloat for a much longer time. First the person should try to swallow air into the stomach. After filling the stomach with plenty of air, he should take the deepest inhalation followed by retention. After retaining the breath as much as possible, exhalation should be done slowly.

Pranayama involves conscious rhythmic breathing with retention. Normally we breathe in and breathe out in three to four seconds. With Pranayama, the breathing cycle takes thirty to seventy seconds. Thus with this procedure, respiratory efforts are saved, which in turn benefits vitality. As the span of life is increased, this is a very useful procedure. It is observed that athletes who do heavy exercise with short and quick breathing have comparatively short life spans, irrespective of a beautifully built body and admirable features. This is the case with boxers, weight lifters and wrestlers, who spend much time in excited states of mind with quick and short breathing.

The lotus posture or the posture of Svastikasana give steadiness and relaxation to the entire body. With this kind of posture, there is very little chance for stimuli coming from skeletal muscle. The vertebral column is adjusted in a straight position so that there is minimal stimulation of the adjacent nerves. The neck movements are smoothly restricted and the eyes are closed to minimize stimuli arising from them. Having attained all these for a sustained period of relaxation, the breathing procedure with alternate nostrils follows.

According to Ayurveda, Pranayama is not only the exercise of the lungs but also an exercise for all the hollow organs in the body. The parenchymatous tissue of the lung taxes the circulation when it is in an active stage during normal respiration. With Pranayama it is rendered almost at rest by sustained relaxation. At the same time, the rhythmic contraction and relaxation of the major hollow organs in the abdominal area allows them to throw away sticky waste material that has accumulated in them. Thus indirectly Pranayama has a cleansing effect on all the hollow organs of the body. It also helps the propulsion of Doshas toward the digestive tract.

In Pranayama, rhythm is very important. Due to this rhythm, the lungs as well as other major hollow organs engaged in the process can drive out their waste products and keep themselves clean. If we compare this with low and high tides of the sea, then we will understand why the sea can throw off any material put into it. Lakes, on the other hand, do not have such rhythm, hence everything put in goes to the bottom and remains there as silt. During the rainy season, the rhythm of the sea gets disturbed, hence it cannot throw out all the silt put into it and becomes polluted.

Therefore it is clear that there is a certain relationship between the lungs and the other hollow organs, particularly those responsible for digestion. Similarly if there is rhythm in the contraction and relaxation of the lung parenchymatous tissue, it also helps to get rid of the waste products in them. It is interesting to note that whenever the digestive tract or any hollow organ is filled with excessive fluid, as when we have overeaten, when the bladder is filled with urine, or even when there is excessive fluid in the circulatory channels, as in congestive cardiac failure, there is always dyspnea or difficulty in breathing.

By understanding this, it can be said that the health-promoting effect achieved by Pranayama is not restricted to the lungs alone. If the lungs are kept clean by a process of conscious and rhythmic breathing, other hollow organs can be maintained clean and healthy, and through them the entire body can be cleansed.

ALTERNATE NOSTRIL BREATHING IN AYURVEDIC TREATMENT

First let us consider anatomy according to Yoga. The Pingala Nadi or right subtle nerve channel starts from the right side of the perineum and crosses the vertebral column from left to right at each chakra, ultimately ending in the right nostril. The Ida or left subtle nerve channel starts from the left side and, crossing the vertebral column twice, ends in the left nostril.

The right side of the trunk contains the main organs responsible for digestion — the liver and the larger part of the head of the pancreas. On the other hand, the organs responsible for nourishment — the heart and the stomach — are located on the left side of the trunk, which includes the thoracic duct.

Even though there are two nostrils divided by the nasal septum, the breathing predominent at one time is through one nostril only. Respiration from the right to left nostril normally shifts after a particular period, or according to the environment. Right-nostril breathing is more observed when the environment or body conditions are cool. When the body and outside conditions are comparatively hot, breathing is mainly from the left nostril. Because the right side of the body is predominantly hot, right-nostril breathing compensates for cold. Similarly, because the left side of the body is predominantly cool, left-nostril breathing compensates for heat. The right side of the body predominant in the solar or heat principle is catabolic (stimulating and reducing) in nature, while the left side predominant in the lunar or cold principle is anabolic (building or sedating) in nature.

Therefore, if only left-nostril breathing is continued for a long time it has a cooling effect, while right-nostril breathing alone is heating. Hence patients suffering from cold diseases like obesity, edema, and muscle stiffness should be advised to breathe only through the right nostril. In these patients, the left nostril should be closed by a cotton swab. To start off, this practice should be done for thirty seconds only. It should be increased slowly to two or three minutes at a time.

On the other hand, patients suffering from hot or catabolic diseases like cancer, weight loss due to chronic fevers, improper digestion, and other wasting diseases should be asked to breathe only through the left nostril. This type of breathing is also helpful in patients suffering from paralysis with flaccid muscles.

Left-nostril breathing is also useful in conditions of hyperactivity of the mind including insomnia, restlessness, and nervous agitation. Right-nostril breathing is useful in hypoactive conditions of the mind including sleepiness, dullness, and fatigue.

* * *

YOGA PROCEDURES ACCORDING TO CONSTITUTION

We have already seen that constitution refers to the typology of individuals according to the predominance of the Doshas. This dominance casts its impression on all body structures, various functions, growth requirements, psychological reactions, and so on.

The healthy body demands balancing factors to its constitution. As the different degrees of warmth or cold, wetness or dryness, or heavy or light food may be required by different individuals to maintain health, so too the Yoga procedures for them to follow also have a constitutional bearing. This means that if specific Yoga procedures are followed according to constitution, they will be more beneficial for one's health.

Yoga Procedures for Vata

Vata people require Yoga procedures which will not exhaust them. They should follow Svastikasana, Padmasana, or Sukhasana postures every day. Also useful are Vajrasana and Siddhasana. Postures that allow the major muscle tissue areas restricted action are most useful. To control Vata they should practice meditation in those postures. With the help of meditation the mind can be kept under control, which in turn controls Vata.

They should also practice mainly right-nostril breathing. Inhalation with the right nostril and exhalation with the left nostril every day for ten to fifteen minutes compensates for coldness due to Vata and hence is very beneficial.

As far as possible, they should not carry out the stronger purificatory procedures like Dhouti (though Jala Neti and Trataka are good). For them, enema treatment (Basti) is most useful because it alleviates constipation, their most common complaint.

Yoga Procedures for Pitta

Pitta people have excess hot and warm qualities in their body. To compensate for these they should follow Yoga procedures which create coolness. Shitali inhalation and Sitkari exhalation have this effect.

According to the Yogic understanding of the body, the position of the Sun principle in the body is around the umbilicus, while that of the Moon is around the soft palate in the mouth, where salivary secretions are constantly taking place. It is thought that the Sun with its heat directed upwards functions to reduce the activity of the Moon in the soft palate. Putting the body regularly in Viparitakarini, the shoulder stand (Sarvangasana) or plough pose (Halasana) helps protect the lunar principle from the effects of the solar principle and creates coolness in the body. Due to these postures, the positions of the Sun and the Moon get reversed. This is naturally beneficial for Pitta types.

Pitta people are also benefited by postures which give a slow massage of the liver and spleen area. For this purpose, they should carry out the bow pose (Dhanurasana), cobra pose (Bhujagasana) and fish pose (Matsyasana). These postures allow excess Pitta to be eliminated from the body.

Yoga Procedures for Kapha

Kapha people usually have slow digestion and low metabolism. To stimulate the digestive capacity, procedures having an action on the navel region (where Agni is situated) are very useful. These are Nauli, Agnisara, or Nauli chalana. Purificatory procedures like Neti and Dhouti are especially useful for them. Paschimottasana is the most beneficial of the Yoga postures, as is Yogamudra. Similarly the Ujjayi type of Pranayama, if done regularly, reduces excess Kapha in the body.

APPENDICES

1
MODERN AYURVEDIC
TREATMENT OF OBESITY

Obesity is the most common metabolic disorder of man and one of the oldest documented diseases. In India, as early as 1500 B.C, Charaka described it under "Medoroga" meaning the diseased state (roga) of the adipose tissue (medas). Charaka's description and explanation of the disease and the treatment methods he prescribes for it remain valid today. Through Charaka, Ayurveda has this to say about one suffering from this disease:

An individual whose increased adipose and muscle tissue makes his hips, abdomen and breasts pendulous, and whose vitality is much less than his body size should be called one whose fat tissue is diseased (Medorogi) or is obese (Sthula).[1]

The body is the result of nutrition, of what we eat and how we digest it. Charaka says, "The body is the product of food. Disease occurs as the result of faulty nutrition. The distinction between health and disease arises as a result of the difference between the wholesome and unwholesome diet."[2] Yet Ayurveda also recognizes the role of the mind and life-style in creating health or disease. Ayurveda describes the causative factors of obesity as the overeating of foods that are heavy, cold, sweet, and oily or greasy in nature. Non-dietary factors are lack of exercise, sleeping during the day, abstinence from sexual intercourse, lack of mental effort and striving, and hereditary factors.

In studying the factors behind obesity, modern science has tried in many ways to pinpoint the prime cause. Mental and emotional influences on eating patterns as well as cultural influences and socio-economic status all can have an effect. Genetic factors play a role, but their mechanism remains unknown. Estrogen and androgen hormonal balance appears to influence the sites and amount of adipose tissue deposition, since women and children have a higher proportion of subcutaneous fat than men. Only in rare instances of hypothalamic obesity can the etiology be clearly defined in scientific terms. In this regard the holistic Ayurvedic analysis of the condition may prove more useful than a simple biochemical model.

Due to excessive eating of heavy, cold, sweet, and oily foods, derangement of the digested food mass takes place and produces Ama or improperly digested food, which disturbs the process of nutrition in the body. Due to its production, the first tissue of the seven, plasma (Rasa Dhatu), is not properly formed. Instead, the food undergoes fermentation and putrefaction, being retained in the stomach.

This Ama causes the digestive fire in the adipose tissue to be lowered. Due to its depression, pathological adipose tissue is developed instead of normal adipose tissue and blocks the further chain of tissue formation in the bone, marrow, and reproductive tissues. Simultaneously, it affects the tissues prior to the adipose in development, namely the muscle, blood, and plasma. It thus disturbs the proper formation of all tissues.

The accumulated adipose tissue blocks the channels and Vata and finds no place to go except into the stomach. Vata, which plays a key role in the transformation of the tissues, gets disturbed and accumulates in the digestive tract. This agitated Vata or nervous energy stimulates the digestive fire and further increases appetite and thirst. As a consequence, the individual feels more hunger. Eventually any food taken in will be converted into adipose tissue and will further increase appetite and hunger creating a vicious cycle with no easy relief.

Charaka defines the signs and symptoms of obesity as, "Reduction of longevity, premature aging, depression of sexual drive, difficulty in sexual performance, unpleasant body odor, excessive sweating, dyspnea on mild exertion, difficulty breathing, excess hunger, excess thirst, difficulty walking, tiredness, general debility, loss of vitality, and mental confusion."[3]

The life span is shortened owing to the derangement in metabolism, which blocks tissue regeneration and weakens vitality as a whole. The inability to properly form the reproductive tissue impairs sexual function, and menstrual irregularities occur in females. The blocked metabolism and accumulated heaviness eventually cause the mind to become dull or confused and the power of perception to be reduced.

The complications of obesity lead to many diseases. The following are described in Ayurveda as the most common: diabetes, fistula, lipoma, arthritis, oligomenorrhea (scanty menstrual discharge), heart diseases leading to hypertension, hyperacidity, kidney infection, and hyperhidrosis (excessive sweating). Diabetes, fistula, and lipoma occur more in Kapha constitutions. Arthritis is more common in Vata types. Pitta types suffer more from complications like hypertension, hyperacidity, and kidney infections.

MANAGEMENT OF OBESITY: A HOLISTIC APPROACH

Ayurveda recommends a multidimensional approach in the management of obesity. The treatment is planned with consideration of its causative factors on six levels:

- Weakening of the digestive fire or metabolic power in the adipose tissue
- Production of Ama or improperly digested food
- Disturbed Vata or nervous energy
- Blockage of the channels
- Life-style factors
- Preventative measures and rejuvenation (Rasayana)

The vicious cycle which results in obesity must be broken. To raise the metabolic power or digestive fire in the adipose tissue, herbs like guggul and shilajit are used. Ama production is treated by toxin-burning herbs like guggul, shilajit, and catechu. Aggravation of Vata is treated by medicated enemas of the cleansing type (Niruha Basti). Channel blockage is alleviated by fat-reducing (Lekhana) herbs which have a scraping action to open the channels like black pepper, barberry, or the formula Trikatu. Externally, the same channel-cleansing effect is achieved by application of dry herbal powders like calamus. Diet recommendations also consist of food substances having fat-reducing (Lekhana) action. Examples of preventative and rejuvenative herbs for obesity are haritaki or the Triphala formula.

Life-style factors relate primarily to diet and exercise. Diet emphasizing pungent and bitter tastes, which are composed of the light elements of fire, air, and ether, are advocated as they produce lightness in the body. Sweet taste is restricted in the diet as its earth and water elements increase heaviness. A light diet is recommended to provide only the necessary energy and not increase fat deposits. However, Ayurveda does not recommend fasting or crash dieting, as these can further imbalance the metabolism.

Exercise with gradual increase according to the strength of the patient is advised. No strong exertion or straining is recommended by Ayurveda. Exercises are recommended that are simple to perform, do not need mechanical appliances, are not costly, and can be done anywhere.

GENERAL TREATMENT PLAN FOR OBESITY

The three main factors behind obesity must be treated. These are: 1) vitiation of the biological humors (Vata and Kapha), 2) formation of Ama, and 3) suppression of the metabolic power of the adipose tissue. The aim of treatment should be to treat each factor so that a complete cure can be achieved. Hence the treatment plan is in three phases.

I. TREATMENT OF VITIATION OF THE BIOLOGICAL HUMORS
Aggravation of Vata

If the strength of the individual is good, purificatory procedures for Vata, like cleansing enemas (Niruha Basti), should be carried out. After this the patient is subjected to mild oleation and sudation. Only minimum oleation is used for treating obesity, enough to protect the body from the heat of sudation. External oleation can be done with oils containing hot herbs like calamus, ginger, and mustard.

Sudation or sweating methods can be done externally or internally. External sudation can be done by various methods, like whole-body sudation via a steam box. In this method, the patient lies down in a specially made wooden chamber with his neck and head outside it. In the chamber there is a perforated wooden bed on which the patient rests. Below this perforated bed, decoctions of herbs like nirgundi, Dashamula, eucalyptus leaves, or bay leaves are kept slowly boiling. The steam coming from the decoction is used for sudation. Other steam or sweat boxes can be made in which the patient is allowed to sit.

Another convenient method is taking a sauna. However, taking a cold bath or shower immediately after sauna treatment, or swimming in cold water, is not advisable for obese persons. Ideally, sudation with hot and dry air is better than sudation with steam, particularly in intractable cases of obesity.

After sudation, oil enemas (Anuvasana Basti) are given, followed again by cleansing enemas (Niruha Basti). This latter should contain a decoction of Dashamula, honey, salt, additional herbs, and water. Ideally, alternate oil and cleansing enemas should be given.

If the patient does not have the strength for such purification therapies, Vata should be pacified with palliating (Shamana) therapies. Fat-reducing (Lekhana) herbs should be given. Guggul and shilajit are the herbs of choice in this condition. Triphala Guggul, in a dose of 5–6 gms. daily, is excellent.

Aggravation of Kapha

This results from excessive formation of abnormal adipose tissue. The above mentioned fat-reducing herbs also act on vitiated Kapha and remove excess fat from the body. Shilajit should be administered in doses of 1 gm. daily.

For alleviating Kapha, external massage with powders of agaru, calamus, ginger, or mustard should be done. These substances help to remove excess fat deposited under the skin. They also help to restore the elasticity to the skin and improve complexion.

II. TREATMENT OF AMA

Treatment of Ama is done by two methods: administering herbs which destroy Ama (Ama pachana), and increasing the conversion power of Agni by giving substances that stimulate digestion (dipana). The Ayurvedic formula Trikatu (dry ginger, black pepper, and long pepper) is good for both these actions. It should be taken in doses of 1-2 gms., three times a day. Other useful Ama-removing herbs are guduchi, turmeric, cyperus, Triphala, barberry, and gentian.

III. TREATMENT OF FAT METABOLISM

In obesity, although the basic digestive fire (Jatharagni) may be in proper condition, that of the adipose tissue is impaired. Its power to convert fat becomes very low. To increase its power, herbs like Trikatu and guggul should be given in dosages of 1 gm., four times a day. Shilajat can also be given in combination with fat-reducing herbs. Herbs with this action mentioned by Charaka are cyperus, kushtha, barberry, calamus, ativisha, katuka, chitrak, karanj, and turmeric.

Other herbs with similar properties are guggul, arjuna, catechu, camphor, neem, rohitak, shinshipa, apamarga, gotu kola or brahmi, mandukaparni, amalaki, shigru, kantakari, kumbhi, ashwagandha, Triphala, shilajit, and bilwa. These are primarily herbs of pungent, bitter and astringent tastes. Many Western herbs like gentian, golden seal, barberry, burdock, and dandelion have similar properties. Many common spices like ginger, mustard, cayenne, and black pepper are also useful in this regard.

LIFE-STYLE FACTORS IN TREATMENT
Diet

Persons suffering from obesity should use dietary articles like basmati rice, barley, mung beans, red lentils, and horse gram. Honey is the only sweetener that should be used. As far as possible the individual should drink only warm water which is not carbonated. For cooking oils, sesame or mustard oil should be used, with spices like cayenne, turmeric, black pepper, ginger, and rock salt. Vegetables having slightly astringent, bitter, and pungent tastes should be used. Obese persons should take two teaspoons of honey with warm water every day, morning and evening.

Fasting for two days a week, or partial fasting and drinking fruit juices, warm water and honey is good.

Overweight individuals should avoid eating substances prepared with wheat like breads, cakes, and pastries and abstain from dairy products and sweets prepared from milk and sugar (like ice cream). The individual should avoid sweet and salty substances generally, particular white sugar. Non-vegetarian food like fish, shellfish, and heavy meat like pork, beef, and lamb should be totally avoided. Drinking beer and wine and eating food enriched with cheese, butter, and oily substances are similarly not advisable. Cold drinks of all kinds should be avoided.

Exercise

Regular exercise like walking, hiking, horse riding, and swimming is essential. Yogic exercises like Surya Namaskar are very helpful. Suryabhedana — alternate nostril breathing inhaling through the right nostril and exhaling through the left — is also very good. The individual should follow an active pattern of life with rest kept at a minimum, increasing work and mental activity. Staying up late at night is beneficial as well. Too much rest, sleeping during the day (particularly after meals), applying oil to the skin, and bathing with cold water should be avoided.

AYURVEDIC TREATMENT OF OBESITY:
A CONTROLLED CLINICAL TRIAL

Treating obesity with modern medicine is a problem since safe drugs for long-term therapy are not available. Amphetamines have a well-defined abuse potential and drugs like diethylpropion and fenfluramine cause appreciable undesirable side-effects including pulmonary hypertension and depression. Thyroid hormones were once used to treat obesity but are now contraindicated owing to their side-effects. There is a clear need for a safer drug for long-term therapy of obesity. The development of a non-toxic compound with a capacity to hold weight gain in check is much needed.

Herbs described by Ayurveda are comparatively safe and have been used for centuries without such side-effects. Compounds like Triphala guggul, Simhanad guggul, Gokshuradi guggul, and Chandraprabha are claimed to be effective in the treatment of obesity,[4] but their effectiveness has not been tested in controlled clinical trials. Therefore, we undertook a random, double-blind, placebo-controlled clinical trial of these agents in the treatment of obesity.

Ayurvedic Medicines

The four formulas used in the study were obtained from a well-established Ayurvedic company in Poona which has a valid drug license issued by the government of India. The authenticity of each plant and mineral component was established by the quality control laboratory of the company which is also government certified. All tests of identification were carried out by a qualified chemist approved by the Indian Food and Drug Administration.

Clinical Studies

Seventy subjects referred to the obesity clinic were entered in the trial. All were at least 20% in excess of their ideal body weight as defined by the Life Insurance Corporation of India's height and weight recommendations. At the time of entry into the study they had a stable weight and none were taking any drugs to reduce their weight. All were in good health and non-diabetic. None of them had any endocranial disorders. The patients were randomly divided into four groups. Treatment was planned according to Ayurvedic concepts and Triphala guggul was given to all the patients in all groups except the placebo group (Group III). Other medicines given were Gokshuradi guggul (Group I), Sinhanad guggul (Group II), and Chandraprabha vati (Group IV). Individuals in Group 3 received a 250 mg. placebo tablet indistinguishable from the other formulations.

The subjects were interviewed individually with respect to diet and exercise and were suitably advised. Dietary intake was not controlled. The treatment was continued for a period of three months and patients were examined every two weeks. During these visits their body weight, skin thickness, body measurements like waist and hip circumference, blood pressure, temperature, pulse rate, and other clinical examinations were carried out. Subjective findings like increased or decreased appetite, feeling of lightness, sweating, shortness of breath, joint pain, etc., were individually noted. Side-effects of the herbs, if any, were carefully noted down. On entry and at the end of the study, biochemical investigations such as hemogram, urine examinations, serum lipoprotein and cholesterol were noted.

Results

Forty-eight of the seventy subjects completed the study. There were twenty-two dropouts during the course of the study, mainly from the placebo group who felt that they were not getting any benefit from the therapy. Ten subjects from the active groups dropped out due to a variety of reasons including domestic and family problems. A significant weight loss was seen in Groups I, II, and IV compared to the placebo group. However, weight losses among I, II, and IV were not significantly different from each other. None of the patients in the study complained of loss of appetite. Skin fold thickness, circumference of the hips and the waistline were significantly decreased as compared to the placebo group. There was a remarkable reduction in the serum cholesterol and triglyceride levels in subjects receiving the active medicaments as compared to placebo. Subjective improvement like feelings of well- being and lightness, and decreased joint pain appeared to be associated with the non-placebo groups but could not be statistically documented as significant. Minor side-effects like mild diarrhea and nausea were observed (eight in the therapy group and two in the placebo) but did not necessitate withdrawal from the therapy.

Mechanism of Action

Obese patients are notorious defaulters. In this study efforts were made to retain the interest and cooperation of those taking part in the study and therefore very few defaulted. All three Ayurvedic treatment groups resulted in significant losses of weight relative to the placebo groups. It appears that treatment with these herbs can produce a clinically significant weight reduction. The reduction in skin fold thickness and hip and waist circumferences were significantly greater in drug-treated individuals as compared to placebo. The treatment did not produce any significant changes in the pulse rate, body temperature and systolic/diastolic blood pressures, indicating that these drugs do not affect the sympathetic system or thyroid function. Although the food intake was not reduced, the herb therapy appeared not to have an anorexic effect.

The exact mechanism of these herbs cannot be ascertained from this study. Whether these herbs affect lipolysis remains to be studied. These drugs decreased serum cholesterol and at the same time increased the level of H.D.L. cholesterol. Further studies with the individual drug components are warranted.

The most common medicine used in this study was Triphala guggul. It is a traditional formulation consisting of Triphala, a famous mixture of the three myrobalans (haritaki, amalaki, and bibhitaki) along with guggul. Guggul is the most common ingredient in the anti-obesity drugs described by Ayurveda. It is closely related to myrrh, which Western herbalists use for similar purposes. Guggul has been extensively studied for its chemistry. A number of steroidal compounds have been isolated in it which have anti-inflammatory capacity. Fraction A, isolated from guggul, was also shown to have anti-hyperlipidemic activity. Although a definite hypothesis could not be drawn as to the nature of the mechanism of action of these drugs, a definite first step has been taken in the documentation of ancient concepts of Ayurveda using modern parameters.

Triphala Guggul has also been found in Ayurvedic studes to reduce serum cholesterol, serum triglycerides, and increases, the levels of H.D.L. cholesterol, which can prevent the atherosclerotic changes in coronary vessels and prevents the ischemic heart diseases.

TREATMENT OF OBESITY ACCORDING TO CONSTITUTION
The authors of this last study have conducted research on obesity over the last three years at various Ayurvedic hospitals in Poona. Patients were classified according to constitution and the complications they were suffering from.

Group I
These patients were of Vata constitution and also suffered from brachial neuritis, gout, arthritis, constipation, and tremors.

Group II
These patients were of Pitta constitution and also suffered from hypertension leading to heart disease, hyperacidity leading to peptic ulcer, excessive menstrual bleeding, anemia, hemorrhoids, and varicose veins.

Group III
These patients were of Kapha constitution and also suffered from edema due to weak kidney, diabetes due to weak pancreas, amenorrhoea, oligomenorrhoea (reduced menstrual flow), atherosclerosis leading to heart disease (like thrombosis in coronary arteries), stones in the kidney or bladder, and sterility.

SPECIFIC REGIMEN
VATA GROUP
Anti-Vata Diet
Wheat, brown rice, cooked onion, and cooked vegetables like spinach, okra, moderate amounts of potatoes, carrots, green peas and radishes; sweeteners like jaggery or molasses; sesame oil and ghee (clarified butter); spices like ginger, asafoetida, turmeric, fennel, cloves, coriander, cumin, and Trikatu; chicken, meat, chicken soup; buttermilk with rock salt; warm water (preferably kept in a copper vessel overnight)

Herbs

Triphala Guggul, Simhanad Guggul, and Yogaraj Guggul

Exercise and Yoga

Regular meditation and chanting mantras like OM were prescribed, with alternate-nostril Pranayama for ten minutes each day in Padmasana (Lotus Posture) or Sukhasana (simple cross-leg sitting posture). Pavanamuktasana was found to be very effective for getting eliminating constipation in these patients

Massage

Regular massage with Narayan oil

PITTA GROUP
Anti-Pitta Diet

Brown rice, wheat, barley, potatoes, cabbage, asparagus, lettuce, mung beans, cucumber (in small quantity), cauliflower; ghee or clarified butter, milk; chicken soup; raw sugar; spices like coriander and turmeric; plenty of fluids at room temperature

Herbs

Triphala Guggul with Arogyavardhini, Chandraprabha, Sutshekhar

Exercise and Yoga

Shoulder stand, Ardhamatsyendrasana, light exercise like walking every day; left-nostril Pranayama (Chandra nadi); meditation and chanting mantras like OM Rama Krishna Hari for ten minutes

Massage

With Chanadabalalaksahadi oil

KAPHA GROUP
Anti-Kapha Diet

Steamed vegetables without oil and salt, juices of carrot and tomato; rice, potatoes, and fruit juices only in small quantities; warm water for drinking

Herbs

Triphala Guggul, Punarnava Guggul, Gokshuradi Guggul

Exercise and Yoga

Daily heavy exercise like brisk walking or running. Yoga postures like Paschimotasana and Neti. Pranayama with right-nostril breathing (Suryabhedena). Chanting of Gayatri mantra

Massage

With hot oils like mustard, Vishagarbha or with powder containing calamus, pulses like horse gram

2
SANSKRIT GLOSSARY
OF AYURVEDA

Agni	fire, particularly the digestive fire
Ajña Chakra	center of command, third eye
Akasha	ether or space
Alochak Pitta	form of Pitta governing vision
Ama	toxic material caused by poor digestion
Amla	sour taste
Ananda	bliss
Anna	food
Annamaya Kosa	food sheath
Annavaha Srotas	digestive system
Anuvasana Basti	oily enema
Apana Vayu	downward moving of the five breaths
Apas	the element of water
Arishta	herbal wine
Artava	menstrual fluid
Artavavaha Srotas	menstrual system
Artha	goal of wealth or possessions
Asana	yoga posture
Asthi	bone
Astanga Hridaya	Ayurvedic text written by Vagbhatta
Atman	inner Self
Avalambak Kapha	form of Kapha in the chest
Avaleha	herbal jelly
Avidya	ignorance
Ayurveda	the spiritual science of life (a supplement to the Vedas or Vedanga)
Bala	bodily strength
Basti	enema therapy (also means bladder)
Bahya Marga	outer disease pathway (skin and blood)
Bhakti Yoga	yoga of devotion
Bhrajak Pitta	form of Pitta governing the complexion
Bhuta	element

Bhutagni	digestive fire governing an element
Bodhak Kapha	form of Kapha giving sense of taste
Brahmacharya	control of sexual energy
Brimhana	tonification therapy
Buddhi	intelligence, principle of discrimination
Chakra	spinal center of energy
Charaka	ancient Ayurvedic author
Charaka Samhita	Charaka's treatise on Ayurveda
Chikitsa	therapy (giving care to)
Daiva Chikitsa	spiritual therapy
Darshana	system of philosophy
Dharana	concentration, attention
Dharma	goal, principle, law of one's nature
Dhatu	tissue element of the body
Dhatvagni	Agni in the tissues
Dhyana	meditation
Dinacarya	daily regimen
Gati	quality of the pulse
Gunas	attributes, prime qualities of nature
Guru	1. quality of heaviness, 2. spiritual teacher
Hatha Yoga	yoga of physical postures
Hridaya	heart
Japa	repetition of mantras
Jatharagni	digestive fire
Jiva	individual soul
Jñana Yoga	yoga of knowledge
Jyotish	Vedic astrology
Kala	nutritional membrane for the tissues
Kama	desire
Kapha	biological water humor
Karma	bondage to action, the cause of rebirth
Karma Yoga	yoga of service
Kashaya	astringent taste
Katu	pungent or spicy taste
Kledak Kapha	form of Kapha governing digestion
Kshatriya	man of political values
Kundalini	serpent fire
Laghu	light (opposite heavy)
Langhana	reducing therapy

Madhyama Marga	middle disease pathway (deep tissue)
Majja	bone marrow and nerve tissue
Mala	waste material of the body, three total
Mamsa	muscle
Manas	mind as principle of thought
Mantra	words of power or sacred sounds
Marana	Ayurvedic preparation of metals and minerals
Marga	pathway of the body
Marma	vital points on the body
Maya	illusion, cosmic creative power
Medas	fat
Moksha	liberation
Mutra	urine
Mutravaha Srotas	urinary system
Nadi	Ayurvedic name for pulse
Nadi Pariksa	examination of pulse
Nasya	nasal administration of therapies
Nirama	condition of humors without products of indigestion
Niruha Basti	cleansing enema
Niyama	right actions or observances in yoga practice
Nyaya	one of the six Indian systems of philosophy
Ojas	primary energy reserve of body and mind
Pachaka Pitta	form of Pitta governing digestion
Pancha Karma	five cleansing actions of vomiting, enemas, purgation, bloodletting, and nasal medications
Pariksha	examination, diagnosis
Patañjali	founder-renovator of the classical Yoga system
Pitta	biological fire humor
Prabhava	special action of herbs
Prajñaparadha	failure of wisdom or intelligence
Prakriti	Primal Nature, natural state, constitution
Prakriti Pariksha	constituional examination
Prana	1. life force or breath in general, 2. mental form of the life force, 3. inward moving of the five breaths or life force in the head
Pranayama	breath control
Prash	Ayurvedic herbal jelly
Pratyahara	control of senses and mind
Purisha	feces
Purishavaha Srotas	excretory system

Purusha	the Original Spirit or inner Self
Raga	attraction
Rajas	the intermediate principle of energy among the three qualities of nature (Gunas)
Rajasic	having the nature of Rajas
Rakta	blood
Raktavaha Srotas	circulatory system (hemoglobin portion)
Rakta Moksha	therapeutic bloodletting
Rañjak Pitta	form of Pitta coloring the blood
Rasa	1. plasma, 2. taste
Rasayana	Rejuvenation
Roga	disease
Ritucharya	seasonal regimen
Sadhak Pitta	form of Pitta governing the brain
Sama	condition of humors with products of indigestion
Samana Vayu	equalizing form of the five breaths
Sankhya	the system of Indian philosophy enumerating the main principles of cosmic evolution used by all systems
Sattva	the higher principle of harmony of the three qualities of nature (Gunas)
Sattvic	having the nature of Sattva
Satya	truth
Satya Buddhi	ascertainment of truth
Shakti	power, energy, power of consciousness
Shamana	palliation therapy
Shita	cool
Shiva	pure being or pure consciousness
Shodana	purification therapy
Shukra	semen, reproductive fluid
Shukravaha Srotas	reproductive system
Siddhi	psychic power
Sleshak Kapha	form of Kapha lubricating the joints
Sleshma	another name for Kapha or phlegm
Snehana	Oleation therapy, oil massage
Sparshana	touch, palpation
Sushruta	ancient Ayurvedic author
Soma	bliss or pleasure principle at work behind mind and senses

Srotas	the different channel systems or physiological systems
Sutra	axiom, used in Vedic teaching
Swastha	health
Swasthya	state of being healthy
Swasthavritta	regime promoting health
Swedana	sudation, steam or sweating therapy
Tail	medicated oil
Tamas	the lower principle of inertia of the three qualities of nature (Gunas)
Tamasic	having the nature of Tamas
Tanmantra	five prime sensory principles (sound, touch, sight, taste, and smell) behind organs and elements
Tantra	medieval yoga traditions emphasizing use of techniques and rituals
Tapas	discipline, self-discipline
Tarpak Kapha	form of Kapha governing the brain and nerves
Tattva	principle of cosmic evolution (24 total)
Tejas	mental fire
Tikta	bitter taste
Udana Vayu	upward moving of the five breaths
Upanishads	ancient Vedantic scriptures of India
Ushna	hot as primary attribute
Vaidya	Ayurvedic doctor
Vagbhatta	Ayurvedic author
Vajikarana	aphrodisiac
Vaisheshika	one of the six systems of Indian philosophy
Vamana	therapeutic vomiting
Vata	biological air humor
Vayas	life span
Vayu	another name for Vata
Vedas	ancient books of knowledge presenting the spiritual science of awareness
Vedanta	culmination of the Vedas in the philosophy of Self-realization
Vijñana	intelligence
Vikriti	disease state, diversification or deviation from nature
Vikriti Pariksa	examination of disease
Vipaka	post-digestive effect of herbs

Virechana	purgation therapy
Virya	energetic effect of herbs as heating or cooling
Vishuddha Chakra	throat chakra
Vyana Vayu	outward moving of the five breaths
Yama	right attitudes in Yoga practice
Yoga	psychophysical practices aimed at Self-knowledge
Yoga Sutras	textbook of Yoga

3
HERB AND MEDICINE
GLOSSARY

First listed is the common name of the herb used in the book, then the botanical name and the Ayurvedic name, if different from the common name.

Abhrak Bhasma	Ayurvedic oxide of mica	
Aconite	Aconitum napellus	Visha
Agnimantha	Clerodendron phlomoides	
Agrimony	Agrimonia eupatoria	
Ajwan	Apium graveolens	Ajamoda
Aloe	Aloe spp.	Kumari
Amalaki	Emblica officinalis	
Anu Tail	Type of medicated sesame oil	
Apamarga	Achyranthes aspera	
Aragwadha	Cassia fistula	
Arjuna	Terminalia arjuna	
Asafoetida	Ferula asafoetida	Hingu
Ashok	Saraca indica	
Ashwagandha	Withania somnifera	
Ashwatta	Ficus religiosa	
Ativisha	Aconitum heterophyllum	
Bakuchi	Psoralea corylifolia	
Bala	Sida cordifolia	
Barberry	Berberis spp.	Daruharidra
Bayberry	Myrica spp.	Katphala
Bhallataka	Semecarpus anacardium	
Bhringaraj	Eclipta alba	
Bhumyamalaki	Pyllanthus niruri	
Bibhitaki	Terminalia belerica	
Bilwa	Aegle marmelos	
Black Pepper	Piper nigrum	Marich
Brahma Rasayan	herbal jelly mainly consisting of brahmi or gotu kola	
Brahmi	see gotu kola	

Brahmi Oil	Medicated coconut oil prepared mainly with gotu kola	
Brihati	Solanum indicum	
Calamus	Acorus calamus	Vacha
Camphor	Cinnamomum camphora	Karpura
Cardamom	Elettaria cardamomum	Ela
Castor oil	Ricinis communis	Eranda
Catechu	Acacia catechu	Khadir
Cayenne	Capsicum frutescens	Katuvira
Chandanbala-lakshadi Tail	cooling medicated oil consisting mainly of sandalwood and bala	
Chandraprabha	special Ayurvedic formula for weak kidneys	
Chavya	Piper chaba	
Chiretta	Swertia chirata	Kiratatikta
Chitrak	Plumbago zeylonica	
Chyavan Prash	Herbal jelly (prash) mainly consisting of amalaki fruit	
Cinnamon	Cinnamomum zeylonica	Twak
Cinnamon leaf	Cinnamomum tamala	Tejapatra
Citron	Citrus	Bijapura
Cloves	Syzgium aromaticum	Lavanga
Coral Ash	Ayurvedic coral preparation	Prawal Bhasma
Coriander	Coriandrum sativum	Dhanyaka
Cubebs	Piper cubeba	Kankola
Cumin	Cumin cyminum	Jiraka
Cuscuta	Cuscuta reflexa	Amaravalli
Cyperus	Cyperus rotundus	Musta
Dandelion	Taraxacum vulgare	Dughdapheni
Darbha	Imperatu cylindrica	
Datura	Datura alba	Kanaka-dattura
Dill	Anthemum vulgaris	Mishreya
Dhataki	Woodfordia floribunda	
Draksha	Ayurvedic herbal grape wine	
Echinacea	Echinacea angustifolia	
Elecampane	Inula spp.	Pushkaramula
Emetic Nut	Randia dumetorum	Madana-phala
Ephedra	Ephedra spp.	Somalata
Eucalyptus	Eucalyptus globulis	Tailaparni
Fennel	Foeniculum vulgare	Shatapushpa
Fenugreek	Trigonella foenum-graecum	Methi
Flaxseed	Linum usitatissimum	Uma

Gambhari	Gmelina arborea	
Garlic	Allium sativum	Lashuna
Gentian	Gentiana spp.	Trayamana
Ginger	Zingiberis officinalis	Ardra (fresh), Shunthi (dry)
Ginseng	Panax ginseng	Lakshmana
Gokshura	Tribulis terrestris	
Gold Bhasma	Special Ayurvedic mineral preparation made with gold	Suvarna Bhasma
Golden seal	Hydrastis canadensis	
Gotu kola	Centella asiatica	Brahmi
Guduchi	Tinospora cordifoliaalso	also Amrit
Guggul	Commiphora mukul (made with other herbs into various resin preparations called Gugguls)	
Gurmar	Gymena sylvestre	Meshashringi
Harenu	Vitex agnus-castus	
Haritaki	Terminalia chebula	
Holy Basil	Ocimum sanctum	Tulsi
Jambu	Eugenia jambolana	
Jasmine	Jasminum grandiflorum	Jati
Jatamansi	Nardostachys jatamansi	
Jivanti	Dendrobium macrael	
Kakoli	Polygonatum verticillatum	
Kalajaji	Eugenia jambolanum	
Kantakari	Solanum xanthocarpum	
Kapittha	Feronia elephantum	
Kapikacchu	Mucuna pruriens	
Karanj	Pongomia glabra	
Kasa	Saccharum spontaneum	
Katuka	Picrorrhiza kurroa	
Kokilaksha	Asteracantha longifolia	
Kukkutanda Bhasma	Oxide made from peacock's feathers	
Kumbhi	Cares arborea	
Kusha	Desmostachya bipinnata	
Kushta	Saussurea lappa	
Kutaj	Holarrhena antidysenterica	
Lauhadi Rasayana	Rejuvenative medicine made mainly with iron	
Lemon grass	Cymbopogon citratus	Rohisha
Licorice	Glycyzrrhiza spp.	Yashtimadhu

Lodhra	Symplocus racemosus	
Loha Bhasma	specially prepared iron ash	
Long Pepper	Piper longum	Pippali
Lotus	Nelumbo nucifera	Padma
Mahabala	Sida rhombifolia	
Makaradhwaj	Ayurvedic alchemical compound consisting of purified sulphur and mercury along with herbs like camphor, nutmeg, cloves, and Trikatu	
Mandukaparni	Hydrocotyle asiatica	
Manjishta	Rubia cordifolium	
Masha	Phaseolus roxburghii	
Meda	Rosocoea alpinia	
Mrigashringa	Bhasma, Ash or oxide made from deer horn	
Mustard	Brassica alba	Shwetarisha
Myrrh	Commiphora myrrha	Bola
Nagakeshar	Mesua ferrea	
Nagbala	Sida spinosa	
Narayan Tail	Medicated sesame oil made mainly with shatavari	
Neem	Azadiracta indica	Nimbu
Nirgundi	Vitex negundo	
Nishot	ipomoea turpethum	
Nutmeg	Myristica fragrans	Jatiphala
Nux vomica	Strychnos nux-vomica	
Nyagrodha	Ficus bengalensis	
Parisha	Hibiscus populnea	
Pashana bheda	Bergenia ligulata	
Patala	Stereospermum suaveolens	
Patola	Trichosanthes cucumerina	
Pennyroyal	Mentha pulegium	
Peppermint	Mentha piperata	Gamathi phudina
Pinus roxurghii		Sarala
Plaksha	Ficus infectoria	
Pomegranate	Punica granatum	Dadima
Prishniparni	Uraria picta	
Priyangu	Prunus mahaleb	
Psyllium	Plantago psyllium	Snigdhajira
Prasarini	Paedaria foetida	
Punarnava	Boerrhavia diffusa	

Rasna	Pluchea lanceolata	
Rhubarb root	Rheum spp.	Amlavetasa
Rohitak	Tecomella undulata	
Saffron	Crocus sativa	Keshar
Sandalwood	Santalum alba	Chandana
Sarsaparilla	Smilax spp.	Chopchini
Saussurea	Saussurea lappa	Kushta
Senna	Cassia acutifolia	Nripadruma
Shalaparni	Desmodium gangetum	
Shallaki	Boswellia serrata	
Shankhapushpi	Crotalaria verrucosa	
Shatavari	Asparagus racemosus	
Shigru	Moringa concanensis	
Shikai	Acacia concina	
Shilajit	Asphaltum	
Shinshipa	Dalbergia latifolia	
Shirisha	Albizzia lebbek	
Shukti Bhasma	Special Ayurvedic mineral preparation made from mother of pearl	
Shyonaka	Oroxylum indicum	
Silver Bhasma	Rajata Bhasma	
Simhanad Guggul	Guggul made with Triphala, suphur, and castor oil	
Sitopaladi churna	Ayurvedic powder consisting of raw sugar, vamsharochana, long pepper, cinnamon	
Soapnut tree	Sapindus trifoliatus	
Suvarna makshika	Ayurvedic gold preparation	
Suvarna parpatti	Ayurvedic gold preparation	
Trikatu	Ayurvedic formula consisting of dry ginger, black pepper, and long pepper (pippali)	
Triphala	Ayurvedic formula consisting of haritaki, amalaki, and bibhitaki	
Triphala guggul	Medicated resin or guggul made with the formula Triphala	
Trivrit	Ipomoea turpethum	
Turmeric	Curcuma longa	Haridra
Tuverak	Hydnocarpus laurifolia	
Udumbara	Ficus glomerata	
Valerian	Valeriana spp.	Tagara
Vateria indica		Ajakarna

Vetivert	Andropogon muricatus	Ushira
Vetra	Salix caprea	
Violet	Viola spp.	Banafshah
Vamsharochana	Bambusa arundinacea	
Vidanga	Embelia ribes	
Vidari	Pueraria tuberosa	
White musali	Asparagus adscendens	Shveta musali
Wintergreen	Gaultheria procumbens	Gandapura
Yavani	Trachyspermum ammi	
Yogaraj Guggul	Guggul formula particularly useful for arthritis	

4
NOTES

1. AYURVEDA, THE SCIENCE OF LIFE

1. The period of the Vedas dates back to 4000 BC. See *Orion or the Arctic Home in the Vedas*, B.G. Tilak; and *Gods, Sages and Kings: Vedic Secrets of Ancient Civilization*, D. Frawley.
2. *Charaka Samhita* (Shree Gulabkunverba Ayurvedic Society: Jamnagar, India, 1949)
3. *Sushruta Samhita* (Nirnayasagar Press: Bombay, India, 1948)
4. *Ashtanga Hridaya* (Nirnayasagar Press: Bombay, India, 1948)
5. *Madhava Nidana* (Chaukhamba: Varanasi, India)
6. *Sharanghdara Samhita* (Chaukhamba: Varanasi, India)
7. *Bhava Prakasha* (Chaukhamba: Varanasi, India)
8. *Ayurveda Itihasa, Parichaya*, Prof. Subhash Ranade and G.R. Paranjape (Anmol Prakashan: Poona, India, 1984)

4. THE AYURVEDIC APPROACH TO HEALTH

1. See Vagbhatta, *Ashtanga Hridaya*, Sh. Ch.3 and *Charaka Samhita*, Vimana Sthana, Ch. 8/116; Sharira Sthana, Ch. 8/52; and Sutra Sthana, Ch. 27/18-19.
2. *Charaka Samhita*, Sharira Sthana 8/51.
3. *Charaka Samhita*, Indriya Sthana 1/3.

7. THE DISEASE PROCESS ACCORDING TO AYURVEDA

1. *Charaka Samhita*, Sutra Sthana, 18.42-44.

12. YOGA AND AYURVEDA

1. *Hatha Yoga Pradipika.* 2/65.
2. *Shiva Samhita* 3/90, 94; 4/49 to 54; 5/65, or *Hatha Yoga Pradipika*, Jyotsna commentary, 7/52, 3/84, 3/86, 3/97, 3/99, and 4/98.
3. *Hatha Yoga Pradipika*, 1/1.

1. APPENDIX (OBESITY)

1. *Charaka Samhita,* Sutra Sthana, 21/9.
2. *Charaka Samhita,* Sutra Sthana, 28/45.
3. *Charaka Samhita,* Sutra Sthana, 21/4.
4. *Sharangdhar Samhita,* 1084.

5
BIBLIOGRAPHY

Caraka. *Caraka Samhita*. Varanasi, India: Chowkhamba Sanskrit Series, 1976.

Dash, Bhagavan. *Alchemy and Metallic Medicines in Ayurveda*. New Delhi, India: Concept Publishing, 1986.

Dash, Bhagavan. *Concept of Agni in Ayurveda*. Varanasi, India: Chowkhamba Sanskrit Series, 1971.

Dash, Bhagavan and Manfred Junius. *A Handbook of Ayurveda*. New Delhi, India: Concept Publishing, 1983.

Dwarakanath, Dr. C.D.. *Introduction to Kayachikitsa*. Varanasi, India: Chaukhambha Orientalia, 1986.

Frawley, Dr. David. *Ayurvedic Healing, A Comprehensive Guide*. Salt Lake City, Utah: Passage Press, 1989.

Frawley, Dr. David and Dr. Vasant Lad. *The Yoga of Herbs*. Santa Fe, New Mexico: Lotus Press, 1986.

Lad, Dr. Vasant. *Ayurveda, The Science of Self-healing*. Santa Fe, New Mexico: Lotus Press, 1984.

Lele, Dr. R.D.. *Ayurveda and Modern Medicine*. Bombay, India: Bharatiya Vidya Bhavan, 1986.

Morningstar, Amadea. *The Ayurvedic Cookbook*. Santa Fe, New Mexico: Lotus Press, 1990.

Murthy, K.R. Srikanta. *Clinical Methods in Ayurveda*. Varanasi, India: Chaukhambha Orientalia, 1983.

Nadkarni. *Indian Materia Medica*. Bombay, India: Popular Prakashan, 1976.

Ranade, Dr. Subhash and Dr. B.K. Patwardhan. *Handbook of Research Methods*. Poona, India: Ammol Publications, 1989.

Savnur, H.V.. *Ayurvedic Materia Medica*. Delhi, India: Indian Books Centre, 1984.

Sushruta. *Sushruta Samhita*. Varanasi, India: Chowkhamba Sankskrit Series, 1981.

Svobodha, Dr. Robert. *Prakruti, Your Ayurvedic Constitution*. Albuquerque, New Mexico: Geocom Ltd., 1988.

Thakur, C.G.. *Ayurveda, The Indian Art and Science of Medicine.* New York, New York: C.G.A.S.I. publications, 1981.

Tierra, Michael. *The Way of Herbs.* New York: Simon and Schuster, 1983.

Tierra, Michael. *Planetary Herbology.* Santa Fe, New Mexico: Lotus Press, 1988.

Udupa, K.N. and R.H. Singh. *Science and Philosophy of Indian Medicine.* Nagpur, India: Shree Baidyanath Ayurved Bhawan Ltd., 1978.

Vagbhatta. *Ashtanga Hridaya.* (Sanskrit only)

Index

BIODATA

Dr. Subhash Ranade had his B.A.M.& S. from Poona University in 1962 and his M.A.Sc. in 1973. He is a Fellow of the National Academy of Indian Medicine (Varanasi) and Ph.D. He has lectured on Ayurveda in many conferences in Germany, Italy, and the United States. He is a member of various Ayurvedic coucils, schools, and associations in Italy, Japan, Australia, Germany, and the United States. He has given many radio and television programs on Ayurveda in India and has had a regular program on Ayurveda on Bombay television since 1980.

Dr. Ranade has written hundreds of articles on Ayurveda for various publications in India and abroad. He is the author of over thirty-five books on Ayurveda, including reference books for Ayurveda Courses and manuals for the treatment of common diseases. He has more than 20 years of teaching experience in Ayurveda from undergraduate to post-graduate levels.

He is currently the director of the Interdisciplinary School of Ayurvedic Medicine of the University of Poona and Principal of the Ashtanga Ayurveda College also in Poona.

BOOKS OF RELATED INTEREST

The Astrology of the Seers
A Guide to Vedic Astrology by David Frawley
    ISBN 1-878423-05-3   342 pp. $18.95
Ayurvedic Healing
A Comprehensive Guide by David Frawley
    ISBN 1-878423-05-3   342 pp. $18.95
From the River of Heaven
Hindu and Vedic Knowledge for the Modern Age by David Frawley
    ISBN 1-878423-01-1   180 pp. $12.95
Gods, Sages and Kings
Vedic Secrets of Ancient Civilization by David Frawley
    ISBN 1-878423-08-8   396 pp. $19.95
Beyond the Mind
by David Frawley
    ISBN 1-878423-14-2   180 pp. $12.95
Wisdom of the Ancient Seers
Mantras of the *Rig Veda*
by David Frawley
    ISBN 1-878423-16-9   275 pp. $14.95
Myths and Symbols of Vedic Astrology by Bepin Behari
    ISBN 1-878423-06-1   278 pp. $14.95
Fundamentals of Vedic Astrology
Vedic Astrologer's Handbook, Volume I by Bepin Behari
    ISBN 1-878423-09-6   280 pp. $14.95
Planets in the Signs and Houses
Vedic Astrologer's Handbook, Volume II by Bepin Behari
    ISBN 1-878423-10-X   258 pp. $14.95
Aspects in Vedic Astrology
by Pandit Gopesh Kumar Ojha and Pandit Ashutosh Ojha
    ISBN 1-878423-15-0   181 pp. $13.95
Astrological Healing Gems by Shivaji Bhattacharjee
    ISBN 1-878423-07-X   128 pp. $7.95
Interacting With Society
Life Strategies Series by Edward F. Tarabilda
    ISBN 1-878423-03-7   176 pp. $7.95
Happy, Healthful Longevity
Life Strategies Series by Edward F. Tarabilda
    ISBN 1-878423-02-9   160 pp. $7.95
The Spiritual Quest
Life Strategies Series by Edward F. Tarabilda
    ISBN 1-87842 3-04-5   125 pp. $7.95